seeking

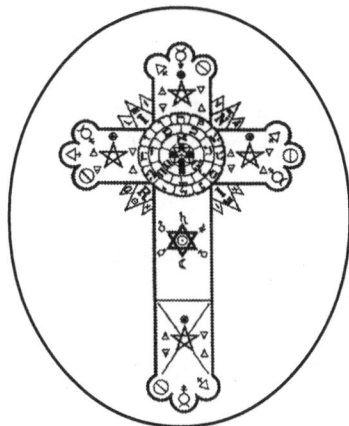

THE
ALCHEMICAL
CURE FOR
CANCER

Miguel F. Brooks, B.Sc., Ph.D., F.R.C.

With a foreword by Professor the Honourable
Errol Y. St. A. Morrison
Pro Vice Chancellor and Dean,
University of the West Indies

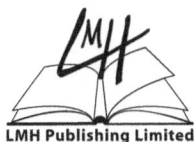

LMH Publishing Limited

Cover Design: Errol Rhule
Book Design, Layout & Typeset: Michelle Mitchell, PAGE Design Services

Published by: LMH Publishing Limited
7 Norman Road,
LOJ Industrial Complex,
Building 10,
Kingston C.S.O., Jamaica.
Tel: 876-938-0005; 938-0712
Fax: 876-759-8752
Email: lmhbookpublishing@cwjamaica.com
Website: www.lmhpublishingjamaica.com

Printed in the U.S.A.   ISBN   976-8184-35-3

Warning

The author does not directly or indirectly diagnose, dispense medical advice or prescribe the use of Alchemical or Occult methods, herbs or any other substance as a form of treatment without medical approval. The intent is only to offer information. In the event you use this information without your doctor's approval, you are prescribing for yourself, which is your right, but the publisher and author assume no responsibility.

Dedication

To my friend Dr. Héctor Velarde Valdés, the indomitable Modern Alchemist who kept his spirit strong while in the depths of Hell. Your loving gift of timeless wisdom lives on, as we continue seeking that which others conceal...

Acknowledgements

My sincere gratitude goes out to all those who offered encouraging words and emotional and moral support in the face of multiple staggering obstacles and challenges confronted in the preparation of this work.

Special thanks to the Hon. Mr. Mike Henry, CD, M.P., my fearless publisher and mentor, for his abiding faith in me and for his stubborn loyalty. The dauntless, unwavering assistance and guidance that he gave me through many years of plodding toil and labour, made it all possible.

I remain eternally grateful to my friend Dr. Carlton Fraser, M.D. who was there from the beginning; to Miss Beverley Williams for her insightful, critical review of the early manuscript drafts, and to Dr. W. Val Chambers, Ph.D. for his most valuable suggestions and contribution.

I am also profoundly indebted to Dr. Amable Thaureaux-Bataille, M.D. and to Dr. Walter E. Davis, M.D. for their precious Medical and Alchemical review opinions and timely advice.

The heavy burden of editorial and pre and post-production tasks were ably carried out by Miss Dawn Chambers, Manager, LMH Publishing, Mr. Bindley Sangster, Editorial and Production Manager, and their technical teams.

Your kind help and tireless efforts were not fruitless. *Thanks!*

M.F.B.

Contents

Foreword

"SEEKING THE ALCHEMICAL CURE FOR CANCER" is a gripping tale of serendipity juxtaposed with misfortune, despair and hope. The collegial kinsmanship and bonding which develops between the Jamaican author and the spectrum of individuals encountered; the transfer of knowledge and the regrouping of like minds speak to history in evolution within the context of a wider historical setting.

The details of life in a Jamaican prison; the revolutionary armies of Colombia and Bolivia; the tracing back of prehistorical times and the explanations of various alchemical practices are vivid treats to a panoramic roller-coaster of events, which all have a link to the theme and explanation of the evolution of Alchemy. The setting in which this scientific search is posited is wildly unique and in like manner, the proposed revitalisation of the 'drug' trade. The proposed mechanism of action of this alchemical compound is in keeping with cutting edge thinking as to the possible role of immunotherapy in the treatment of immuno-compromised states such as cancers, HIV/AIDS etc.

This apart, the writer's style is engaging, the research thorough and probing, both historically and in scientific depth. This is a compelling tome, thrilling from cover to cover and completely sates the appetite for information on a variety of issues; freemasonry, narcotrafficking, the Black Death, the Catholic Inquisition and more.

Once you begin, you will read on.

Thoroughly interesting!

Let me remind the author and his regrouped team of the Chinese Proverb:

> *'Man who says it can't be done*
> *Must not interrupt man doing it!'*

Best of luck!

Errol Y. St. A. Morrison, *OJ, MD, PhD, FRCP (Glasg.), FACP, FRSM (UK)*

Professor the Honourable Errol Y. St. A. Morrison is currently
   - Pro Vice Chancellor and Dean, School for Graduate Studies & Research
      (University of the West Indies)
   - Professor of Biochemistry and Endocrinology (U.W.I.)
   - He is also Co-Founder & honorary Life President, Diabetes Association of Jamaica

Introduction

*F*or over twelve years I had been burdened with the knowledge of the existence of a possible natural overall cure for the scourge of Cancer, but, apart from my initial disbelief, I had also not settled in my mind just what to do about this extraordinary information.

During this long period, I had on several instances abandoned and even forgotten the whole matter, relegating it to the realm of a mere intellectual curiosity, or at best, to some kind of allegory, employing the imagery of disease and cure to outline what was in reality a moral or idealistic 'spiritual' cure and restoration of man's character.

My original contact with the sources revealing this secret Alchemical cure for Cancer, came through veiled and enigmatic intimations that I encountered in the course of my Philosophical and Esoteric studies. Further and rather extensive corroboration of the fact that there was indeed in antiquity, a cure for Cancer and many other serious illnesses, came during lengthy research I conducted on the Ark of the Covenant and which culminated in the publication of the definitive Modern English language translation of *KEBRA NAGAST* (The Glory of Kings), the sacred book of Ethiopia.

It was, however, my providential and mysterious meeting with Doctor Héctor Valdés, and the friendship we forged, that brought the most dramatic and persuasive evidence to the effect that the ancients were in fact able to cure Cancer, and had indeed done so frequently. Héctor Valdés provided me with irrefutable proof that confirmed not only the validity of rare accounts in the annals of Occult Medicine, but also the astounding revelation that the Alchemical cure for Cancer had been successfully replicated during the past two decades in South America.

All this had remained dormant in my mind for many years, subsumed to the abundance of overwhelming cares, to the common assail of daily routine, and to the stresses of modern life. Yet, periodically, the occasional rare data would arrive, adding to the growing body of relevant information that I had been accumulating.

Then, around four years ago I experienced some strange promptings, suggesting to me that I should 'do something' about all the detailed clinical, technical and historical data in my possession. But, it was the disturbing frequency of Cancer-caused deaths among friends, acquaintances, and the unknown ones we read about in the press making up the frightening statistics worldwide, which finally convinced me that I could not continue to keep to myself, that which might well hold the solution to one of mankind's deadliest enemy, Cancer.

My first instinct told me that I should attempt a replication of the South American clinical experience, as the natural sources for obtaining the biological extracts used, are readily and abundantly available in Jamaica, and the procedural methodology is well defined and fully documented. To this end a work team led by Medical Director Dr. Carlton 'Pee Wee' Fraser, M.D. was organised, and a remote site at an old slavery-days plantation, complete with a Great House and dungeons for slaves, was identified. These facilities were placed at our disposal by the sympathetic owner of the thousand-acre holding.

The project would conduct extraction of the biological substance 'in situ', effect the required basic processing, and go on to the clinical assessment, for which a number of terminally ill cases were available. We contacted the Sloan Kettering Memorial Center, the Jamaica Cancer Society, the La Jolla Cancer Research Institute, the American Cancer Society and several other international Cancer Research Institutions, seeking to share the knowledge we have, and inviting them to explore with us the possibility of some kind of collaborative effort in reconfirming the efficacy and safety of the Alchemical cure for Cancer. They did not respond to, or even acknowledge our communications.

Early in 1988 I decided to write a detailed account of all aspects of this ancient Alchemical cure for Cancer, along with all the considerable body of Arcane and Esoteric data, on the exquisite art of the old Alchemists and practitioners of Occult Medicine accumulated through many years of painstaking research. I had also decided to chronicle in plain, straightforward narrative, all relevant aspects and circumstances surrounding the baffling events leading to my fateful meeting with Dr. Valdés in Kingston, Jamaica.

I have earnestly tried to document here, every matter, event or data, which I believe to be germane to a true appreciation of the import of a modern rediscovery of the Alchemical cure for Cancer. And, although this work does not purport to be a scientific or medical report, I do hope that in it will be found sufficient information to stimulate a comprehensive and thorough investigation by the international Cancer research fraternity, whom, with the extensive facilities and resources at their disposal, can either confirm or refute the historical and the recent clinical evidence, that there is in certain natural biological substances, the answer to man's age-old quest in search of a cancer cure.

Not all data is contained herein. The technical information on methods of substance extraction, sterilization, as well as procedural methodology on clinical application and assessment, are given in the *'Manual of Substance Preparation and Clinical Procedures'* which is now being edited and reviewed. It will be made available to any research institute engaged in evaluating BRM's (Biological Response Modifiers), who would be willing to conduct the required series of investigations and Clinical Studies on the Alchemical claims of having discovered a reliable, natural and safe cure for most forms of Cancer.

It is my fervent hope that these efforts will begin soon, or at least before our forests and woodlands, the fauna and flora so graciously bequeathed to us by the Creator, is finally and hopelessly obliterated by destructive man seeking to satisfy his immediate greed, as he continues in blissful ignorance, ravishing and denuding the earth of its most precious patrimony.

SEEKING: The Alchemical Cure for Cancer, is the testimony of one man; that which evolves from it will be the Legacy of this generation unto those not yet born.

M. F. BROOKS

Chapter 1

The Biochemist

*T*hey had received the call at about noon, then at exactly one o'clock the message was relayed to me. There was a 'Spanish man' who needed some help from an interpreter, and once more the parish priest at Saint Anne's Church in Kingston had directed them to me. In the last two years many Latin Americans had been arrested in Jamaica on drug trafficking charges; most of them were caught aboard luxury yachts, others on fairly small fishing boats which they navigate across the Caribbean sea from as far south as the Colombian coast unto Jamaican waters.

I agreed to render some assistance, as I've usually done, to a fellow Latin compatriot in need, as I not only had a deep seated sense of empathy and even some solidarity towards these 'paisanos', but I also welcomed the opportunity to get first hand impressions of the current situation back home.

Over the years I had met quite a few of these adventurous fellows, among them were Hondurans, Colombians, Cubans, Nicaraguans and Mexicans. Most of them were lower-echelon couriers and conveyors of illicit drugs for a number of fairly large organizations. During the 1980's most of them were caught in the

Cayman Islands and sent to Jamaican prisons for safekeeping under the terms of an agreement between the two British territories.

It was evident that the Caribbean was being used by the South American drug cartels as a convenient trans-shipment zone to move huge quantities of Cocaine to Europe and North America, and so there was a nervous sense of alertness in the area directed especially towards Latin American travellers, manifested in the pathetic paranoia of so many small-island governments eagerly taking orders from sundry US drug enforcement agents, and shamelessly giving up whatever semblance of sovereignty they had.

By late evening on that same day I went to the office of the Superintendent of the General Penitentiary, Jamaica's largest maximum security prison on Tower street in the crime-infested inner city area of downtown Kingston, to await the arrival of another 'special prisoner'. Some ten minutes later he arrived and was escorted to the office where three officers and myself were seated around a large working table.

I was surprised to see that he had two enormous suitcases and an attache-case plus a travelling bag with him. Short, stocky and barrel-chested, with the typical features of the Andean Incas, he exuded a quiet dignity and poise that indicated his upper middle class status, while his deference and politeness revealed a cultured upbringing and education.

Looking dejected and miserable, he quickly brightened up when I introduced myself and explained that I was assigned to act as his interpreter and guide, since his knowledge of English was limited. This he corrected, saying that he only spoke Spanish and Quechua, the Inca dialect. He knew not a word of English.

After responding to a few routine questions from the officers, I made arrangements for him to be located comfortably at the prison's hospital where a number of other Spanish-speaking prisoners were, and where he would be able to keep all of his personal things too. A few days later we met again, and in numerous subsequent occasions when we had long and most interesting conversations, I came to learn the extraordinary story of

2

this mysterious gentleman.

He was Doctor Héctor Velarde Valdés, a Bolivian biochemist from the jungle town of Santa Cruz where he operated his own biomedical laboratory and a small neon sign enterprise along with his son. At that time in 1982, he was around 53 years old. And this distinguished looking, bespectacled South American scientist was arrested at the Norman Manley International Airport where over one kilogram of pure cocaine was found professionally built into the thick soles of his platform shoes.

Dr. Hector Valdés was really in transit through Jamaica on his way to Miami. He was travelling from Santa Cruz, Bolivia through Lima, Perú, and should have rendezvous with a tall American known only as 'Douglas' at a guest house in the Jamaican resort of Negril. The American would have taken the platform shoes from him in exchange for U.S. $52,000.00 and he would then be on his way to Miami. But something had gone terribly wrong, and in retrospect he now realized what had really happened.

It was his son's wife, Deyanira Velarde, the only one in the family who knew English and who had established the link with 'Douglas' in Negril. Along with her young husband, Julio Velarde, they had already made three trips to Jamaica as tourists and successfully transacted business which provided the capital to establish the neon sign outfit and also allowed Dr. Valdés to fully equip his biomedical laboratory. Generally, things went along pretty well for them, in spite of the incipient alcoholism of young Julio Velarde, who at 24 years of age was under the bewitching sway of the knowing and experienced Deyanira and her crafty sluttishness which she used in all the wisdom of her feminine wiles, to advance the welfare of her side of the family.

They were citizens of Santa Cruz, the wealthy town in the heart of Bolivia's coca growing region, where vast fortunes are made by the cheap purchase of PBC (Pasta básica de cocaína/cocaine base) or from the bitter crystalline alkaloid processed from the coca leaves, to be sold in the US or Europe at greater profit than mined gold. Entire mountain sides and large stretches of flatland in the high plains were cultivated by the peasantry with

3

the South American shrub, whose leaves are chewed by natives to impart endurance.

The region around Santa Cruz was the undisputed domain of the legendary 'drug baron' José Raul Gómez, the one who had offered to pay off Bolivia's 6.8 billion dollar external debt in exchange for official guarantees that would allow his fleet of airplanes to move freely from their jungle bases. The economy of the whole region depends on coca leaves cultivation and processing, and the palatial residences with their gaudy luxury along with the showy display of ostentatious living, stand as testimony to the easy wealth of the 'coca-dollar' entrepreneurs of Santa Cruz.

But the tensions within the Velarde Valdés family were deepening, as Deyanira had become intimate with the young scion of a leading family in high society. Violent disputes between herself and her young husband Julio had taken ominous overtones, and neither of them at that time knew that her new lover, Melesio Mieres, was an undercover agent for the US Drug Enforcement Agency. Deyanira had moved out of the Valdés residence after a particularly nasty fight with Julio, and had along with her young daughter gone to live with Melesio at his ranch outside of Santa Cruz.

Julio Velarde and his father Dr. Hector Valdés pondered over what to do next, since Deyanira was the principal contact and negotiator with 'Douglas' in English-speaking Jamaica. But then, Julio did travel with her on each journey and he knew the American and also knew the guest house in Negril where he could be found. They decided then that Julio and his father would make the trip to Jamaica, since they already had almost three kilos of refined cocaine at hand.

A little over one kilogram of the crystalline white powder was taken to the 'old man', the master shoemaker who would construct the pair of platform shoes with its hollowed-out thick soles packed with the cocaine. The 'old man' had developed his skill to such a degree of perfection that the finished shoes looked like factory-issued ones, complete with brand tag and all.

During the decade of the eighties, the Soviet airline Aeroflot had scheduled flights once a week from Lima, Perú to Kingston, Jamaica. Both, father and son quietly left Santa Cruz for Lima where they would remain for two days awaiting the Aeroflot flight to Jamaica. While they were ensconced at a hotel in the Peruvian capital, young Julio telephoned a friend back in Santa Cruz, a mistake that would prove to be their undoing, because word reached his estranged wife Deyanira that Julio was in Lima, instantly alerting her that he was on his way to Jamaica with merchandise for the American, Douglas. She of course, shared this bit of information with her paramour Melesio who soon after passed it on to his DEA manager.

When they had embarked the Aeroflot flight in Lima, they became alarmed by the fact that Julio was singled out for a particularly detailed search of his baggage and his person, then allowed to go on the flight. It was then, during the fairly long journey to Kingston that Julio disclosed to his father that he had called a friend in Santa Cruz from their hotel in Lima. They then saw how and from whence the treachery had come. Deyanira knew that Julio was travelling to Jamaica; what she did not know what that his father Dr. Hector Valdés was also on the flight, and was the one wearing the loaded shoes.

Upon realizing that Julio's father was also on that flight, the Jamaican authorities were informed and Dr. Hector Valdés was held at the airport as he was going through immigration processing. His baggage was not searched, but he was requested to take off his shoes which a police officer immediately cut with a knife disclosing its stuffing of white powdery substance. Julio was allowed to pass through unhindered.

Dr. Valdés was speedily arraigned before the court and his state-appointed attorney advised him to plead guilty since he had no defense. He was given a two year sentence plus a fine of J$169,000.00 which if not paid would mean another year of added sentence. Julio had returned to Bolivia before the trial had taken place.

All this I had learned from Dr. Valdés in the course of many long conversations we held and by which a close friendship and brotherlike bond gradually developed between us. For he was a highly educated man, cultured and knowledgeable much beyond the scope of his biomedical specialty, and so, our frequent exchanges on a wide variety of topics, were made pleasurable through the medium of the fluid and versatile Spanish language we both mastered.

He related to me in minute detail all matters pertaining to his background, his family life, the affairs of his country, Bolivia, as well as an astounding body of information on rare, exotic medical practices of the Amerindians in the Amazon river basin and in the deep jungles of South America.

And Dr. Valdés was indeed a prominent citizen of Santa Cruz, even a recent past president of the Lions Club in that locality. But what I did find curious was the fact that he was travelling with his entire personal legacy, documents, photos, diplomas and credentials. To me it appeared as if he brought along every single item of personal value that he possessed. In those huge suitcase there was even some exposed x-ray films and copious medical and scientific notes and files.

As I expressed my amazement at his voluminous baggage, he disclosed the true nature of his trip originally destined to Miami. He was really separating from his wife of twenty-two years, leaving everything behind and heading for the USA to undergo an orthopaedic operation on his knee, to be paid for by the cocaine sale money. He would then return, not to Santa Cruz but to Colombia where he had a sister and other relatives. Finding himself stranded for at least the next two years in a Jamaican prison, he now had no idea how things would resolve themselves nor what he would eventually do, if he did survive the ordeal he was now undergoing.

His immediate priority, however, was to have the fine that was imposed as part of the sentence, paid, so that his total time in captivity be reduced by at least one third. I therefore agreed to telephone his wife in Santa Cruz, Bolivia, inform the family of his current status and the sentence given to him, and to persuade them to arrange for payment of the fine.

It was a lengthy conversation, and a difficult one too, with much histrionics and emotional outbursts on their side. Of course there was the testing preamble by the wife, seeking to establish whether I was truly a friend of Dr. Valdés or merely an opportunist trying to get the money by perhaps ambushing the carrier of the funds or something of the sort. But when I mentioned the names of all family members and other details which could only come from Dr. Valdés himself, they immediately realized that the call was a genuine one. A second call three days after brought the good news that Julio Velarde would be travelling to Jamaica in two weeks time to pay the fine. So, we waited.

Meanwhile, Dr. Valdés was slowly adjusting to the daily routine of Jamaican prison life with its nineteenth century colonial rules set in the medieval dungeon-like fortress, the walls of which were undoubtedly built under the lash of slavery. The dismal panorama that met his bewildered eyes were like taken straight out of Dante's inferno, with naked denizens parading their skeletal frames in the open courtyards, scavenging for food in the garbage heaps and drinking putrid water from the open sewers and pits in the compound. We both marvelled at how these individuals remained alive, and ascribed their unbelievable survival to a heightened immunity caused by constant exposure to a veritable cocktail of pathogenic microbes. One of those wretched beings was even seen roasting a rat over an open fire at the rear of one of the cell blocks; other 'criminal lunatics' joined him in enjoying their succulent fare.

The sadistic brutality of the prison guards was another of the more amazing facts in the subculture of prison life that Dr. Valdés tried to understand. We rationalized the many instances of wanton savage beatings that were visited upon the destitute and abandoned inmates by their own people, from the perspective of the terrible history of chattel slavery and abject exploitation that the African descendant population of Jamaica underwent for over three hundred years. The 'divide and rule' principle of applied psychology that was used with such devastating efficiency by the

7

British plantocracy, persisted in its lingering effects upon the black populace of the island.

Being in the 'privileged' area of the prison hospital, largely isolated Hector Valdés from the more primitive depredations that were commonplace in Jamaica's notorious General Penitentiary. There at least, he could fraternize with fellow Latin Americans, like the six Colombians who were caught in the Cayman Islands in a yacht, the hull of which was entirely packed with compressed marijuana. There was also the Cuban exile who after ten years of residence in Cayman had become a noted citizen, a prominent contractor-builder who had donated a school to the island's children and was even introduced to Queen Elizabeth during one of her visits there. He had been importing large quantities of Cocaine from Colombia in bags of cement under cover of his building enterprises. He was arrested during a sting operation by US drug agents posing as interested purchasers.

It was a motley collection of unsavory characters, a rogues gallery of ambitious petty traffickers with dreams of making it big in the 'rags to riches' world of the drug cartels and their legendary leaders. Dr. Hector Valdés however, was not the typical drug courier, but due to a peculiar set of circumstances mainly within his family, now found himself duly classified and stigmatized as another one of those 'dangerous' Latin drug traffickers.

Chapter 2

Physician to the King

*E*urope during the Middle Ages was the scene of profound rivalries where personal relations and conflicts assumed great importance, and where the struggle of the church to assert its spiritual and temporal hegemony brought about widespread accusations of magical and spiritistic practices against anyone who would not accept Rome's ecclesiastical dictatorship. For in that dark era in human history, magic was generally defined by the church as the he retical practice of making pacts with the devil and evil spirits.

Many early Christian writers such as Saint Augustine had considered magic to be a relic of paganism, but it was the Papal bull (official pronouncement by the Pope) of 1320 that firmly defined magic as heresy, and the dreaded Inquisition's records make mention of 'Witches Sabbath' (midnight devil worship assembly) and the 'Black Mass' (a mockery of the Roman Catholic Mass) as forms of witchcraft.

The objectives of the centuries-long murderous Catholic Inquisition which resulted in the torture and execution of over sixty million souls in Europe and the Americas, was to maintain Papal suzerainty throughout the world and to keep all forms of magical, occultic and esoteric knowledge out of the hands of the 'common people'.

Within the Royal courts however, the nobles, the wealthy and urban emerging intelligentsia of Spain, Italy and France especially, were heavy users of many forms of the alchemical tradition. And in the religious and cultural intolerance of those days, many reputed alchemists were regarded as evil magicians, acquiring their knowledge by a pact with the devil, probably because much of their knowledge came from Kabbalistic sources (esoteric Jewish mysticism) which was little understood by even most of the leading scientists of the time.

But the European courts of the Medieval and Renaissance era had the highest regard for the rare skill of the alchemical practitioner, and these were in varying degrees under the protection of Princes, Kings and Nobles, who availed themselves of the wide ranging corpus of arcane and esoteric skills possessed by these mysterious sages.

The tradition among the nobility of Europe, in having a resident 'Physician to the King' goes far back in history. He inherits his office from the ancient priests and prophets of old who acted also as principal advisers to the rulers. Their influence upon the affairs of state was great, as these were men with a broad, universal intellect embracing virtually all areas of human learning, and who were often feared for the power and knowledge they commanded.

Their fearsome reputation was also coloured by the frightful activities of the notorious 'poisoners' who were so prevalent among the royal and titled nobles of the Italian principalities. The famous Médici and Borgia families frequently availed themselves of the services of these experts in all manner of deadly herbal and mineral poisons. Catherine of Médici had her personal poisoner dampen the corner edges of her husband's favourite book on falcon-hunting with poison, which pages he always turned with his tongue-moistened finger. Unfortunately, her beloved son handled the book next, dying instantly with it in his hands. Her husband in turn quietly had his poisoner file a sharp splinter on the inner surface of her ring, treated it with another deadly substance which entered her blood stream when the tiny splinter scraped her finger as she slipped on the treated ring, killing her swiftly.

As from the fourteenth century onwards, the most prominent of these alchemists and 'physicians' were under the protection of royalty and the nobility of the day. *They were reputed to have had at their disposal, treatment and cure for every single malady known then.* All their records and notes on experiments, procedures and methods were meticulously guarded through the secretive use of obscure symbology and allergorical terms understood only by themselves and the initiates of the 'Mystery Schools' who were deemed worthy to receive the knowledge.

Then, at the beginning of the sixteenth century, the leading alchemists came under the influence of the occultic Swiss physician Paracelsus (1490-1541) and his many writings on speculative alchemy; later on, the German philosophic mystic Jakob Bohme had a great influence on the directions of alchemical enquiry with his concepts on the 'polarization of empirical reality'. Bohme claimed to have gained in the period of a quarter hour, an empirical and speculative insight that helped him to resolve the leading questions of his day.

From sometime in the twelfth and thirteenth century onwards, the principal quest of the alchemical experimenter, was the search for the "Philosopher's Stone", a mysterious and elusive substance through which the much desired transmutation of base metals into gold could be achieved. This was one of the most closely guarded secrets ever. Tradition holds that the earliest known successful metallic transmutation was achieved in the days of King Solomon, when a large amount of copper was transmuted into pure gold.

And although the School of Alchemy that flourished in Alexandria in the second century BC could prepare white lead or lead carbonate from litharge, arsenic from realgar, and mercury by roasting cinnabar (mercuric sulfide) in a current of air, there is no indication that they achieved or even attempted to achieve a successful transmutation of base metals into gold.

Reference to the process of transmutation does not reappear until around the twelfth century AD along with the concept of an *actuating substance* or element which the alchemists call "The Philosopher's Stone". Of course, many modern writers, perhaps despairing of the plethora of obfuscating symbols, allegories and arcane formulae, succumb to the tempting notion that by 'transmutation' the alchemist meant a sort of transformation of man's character, from the baser and coarser qualities of the crude, undeveloped person, into the higher, elevated and spiritualized individual; an idealized conception of deity through spiritual change.

The fallacy inherent in this rationalization becomes apparent when it is noted that *fire* and intense *heat,* along with the three alchemical elements of Sulphur, Mercury and Salt are physical factors involved in the transmutation process.

And so it was, that in those days, after the death of King Philip I the Handsome, the first Habsburg king of Castile in 1506, his son, the future emperor Charles V succeeded him first in the Netherlands and later on in 1516, also in Spain. There he appointed the preeminent philosopher and acknowledged expert on Occultism, Cornelius Agrippa, as his court secretary and physician. Agrippa was a German Catholic theologian, formerly a professor at Pavia University; as an orator and public advocate at Metz he was denounced for defending an accused witch, and after a lengthy battle with the inquisitor of Cologne was banished from Germany.

His tempestuous career saw him involved in the state affairs of the Europe of his time, and as military entrepreneur in Spain and in Italy, his activities would have a profound effect on the relationship between the major powers of the day. It is claimed that Agrippa had succeeded in obtaining the 'Philosopher's Stone' and had transmuted fourteen tons of lead into gold for emperor Charles V, an event that greatly helped the consolidation and expansion of the empire, and later on even helped in equipping the ill-fated Spanish Armada that was launched against England by his son King Philip II.

Cornelius Agrippa belonged to that manner of men who were given for life unto the meticulous search for the secrets of nature and the hidden or lost oracles of divinity that were once the common patrimony of mortal men, but that through envy, malice and the larceny that resides in the hearts of the children of men, have been lost forever as the ephemeral riches suddenly acquired by fools, which quickly goes away like the early morning dew.

And in the unending quest of the early Alchemists, many occult revelations from the ancient sages of the Orient, from the land of the Aethiops and from the dominions of the Persians, were carefully documented in the language and symbology that was only understood by the initiates and by those adepts who were deemed worthy after rigorous preparation, trials, tests and examinations, to be admitted into the inner sanctum of the enlightened ones.

Fundamental to Alchemical science was the concept that there are four elements which are the innate principles of all material things. These are: Fire, earth, water and air; and these make up in varying proportions every materialization of the visible world, and they are capable of *reciprocal transmutation* with each other.

Hermes Trismegistus, the God Toth of the Egyptians and father of Alchemy, regarded fire as the preeminent transmuting force, for it is in and within all things where it remains hidden and unknown as long as it does not come into an intimate embrace with matter. It is rapidly mobile by its own action, mixing in a peculiarly destructive manner with anything that comes near to it. It is illuminative, transparent and upwardly mobile tending towards the heavens. Independent of the other elements, it does not allow casual or careless inattention, for it will suddenly reduce matter to ashes with a seeming vengeance. Fire is therefore absolute and unique in its nature and action, yet it is innate in all things; in the rock when struck with the edge of the sword or a steel instrument, in the earth when dug deep enough, in water at many thermal springs, and in air which becomes hot and feeds the flame in intimate combustion... It is therefore present in animals, plants and everything that lives, for they are alive only because of the fire which is within them.

13

And as fire is the animating principle of all living things, water which is its antagonic opposite is no less potent and fundamental, for no living being survives without it. The seminal virtue of all living things resides in water, for none can reproduce without it, and even spiritual rebirth is impossible without water, as the Christ testified unto Nicodemus. Thus, Thales, Plini and Hesiod regarded water as the primeval or first element which controls the others since it covers the earth, extinguishes fire, it goes up and mixes with air where, upon becoming clouds dominates the firmament, and falling upon the earth germinates all that the earth can produce.

Among the ancients, waters with special virtues were well known, such as those of the river Hammon which freezes over at midday yet becomes warm in the morning and evenings; or those waters of a river of the Circassians which turns the entrails hard as stone if drunk and whatever it touches it makes to become as tough as marble. Then in ancient Sybaris in southern Italy, certain spring waters makes the hair of those who drink thereof, golden or amber colour. Or those waters of the lake of Ethiopia which when drunk makes one furious or cause deliriums and stupors.

As Court Secretary and Physician to the King, Cornelius Agrippa had at his disposal a vast quantum of the excellency of human knowledge from many lands that was available in his days. Early in his career he had decided to make it his life's mission and principal endeavour, to document and chronicle the accumulated wisdom of the ages in the fields of Arcane and Mundane Sciences, Medical Arts, and the form of Jewish Occultism known as Kabbalah, or the Jewish Metaphysics of remote antiquity by which these ancient sages explained the universe and its creation.

And the body of human knowledge that had survived countless destructive campaigns of the angry, illiterate and ignorant zealots who were instigated by an intolerant Church and superstitious rulers under her sway, was truly enormous. Much of this had already been lost permanently, but what survived carried with it the rubric of antiquity and the emphatic persistence of those great discoveries that refuse to be obliterated from the annals of mankind.

There is one concept that was evermost present in the minds of all practitioners of the Alchemical arts, which they summed up in the well-known dictum, "As above, so below." Meaning that, as the mechanism of the heavens function under specific laws, so too the modes of material nature here on earth function and are governed by the same principles and laws. They were thus, well aware that all things in the material world are possessed by occult virtues from on high, and that by adhering to certain specific procedures, these occult virtues are susceptible to man's control, manipulation and practical use.

They believed these 'virtues' to originate in the idea or 'creative word' that brought material things into existence, so that, there is a virtue and an admirable power in each herb, in each stone, in each animal, and a corresponding stronger virtue or power in its original idea or concept in the heavens among the celestial bodies.

The occultic concept holds that these virtues or powers are manifested here on earth in concentrated forms in various animals, plants or minerals-stones or in gems, even in certain parts of the human body. And so, it was well known among the adepts of medieval Europe, that the freshly extracted heart of an owl or of a swallow or a beaver, when attached by a scarlet ribbon unto a man's right arm, will stimulate memory, imagination and discernment and also the powers of prognostication or divination. Democritus reveals that the tongue of a toad extracted from the live amphibian that is released unharmed, when placed upon the left breast of a sleeping woman, will cause her to speak while asleep, and she will answer truthfully to any question asked of her while it is in place. He also taught that the tongue of a Chameleon, taken from the live reptile, will ensure favorable judicial outcome, and is also useful for smooth birth delivery when kept on the outside, but very near to, the abode of a laboring woman. It must not, however, be introduced to the premises, for opposite negative effects will ensue.

Those who wish to awaken the fiery passions of love must seek the virtues that reside in the venereal or reproductive organs of the dove, the turtledove, or the swallow, taken when these birds are in a state of excitation; having these on one's person will surely attract intensely the desires of the opposite sex. In like manner, for acquiring a noted boldness and fearlessness, similar use must be made of the eyes, heart or forehead of a lion or a rooster, since the occult virtues of boldness resides therein.

And for these reasons it is known that the kings of Persia routinely provided their ambassadors with the herb *Latax* to ensure that all of their needs will be provided for. Likewise the herb *Sparta* or *Tartary* when placed in the mouth, will allow the person to go for twelve days without food or drink. And the liver of the same Chameleon, when burnt with fire at its tips, will instantly cause lightning, thunder and rains, but its head and neck when burnt on firewood will at once stop the rains. And all these things will surely manifest because of the occult virtue that is immanent in all things; as will be observed with he who carries around his thumb the tongue of a dog dipped in white lime and wrapped with the leaf called 'dog tongue', that no dog nearby is able to bark; and dogs instantly flee from anyone who carries with him the desiccated heart of a dog.

All of the exquisite art of the Alchemist and of the practitioners of Occult Medicine, was not available to the common folk in medieval Europe, but exclusively to royalty and the nobility of those days. For, the accomplished Alchemist usually became a virtual prisoner or a captive in a golden cage, where his rare knowledge and talents were to benefit exclusively the monarch and his court.

The Romans had learnt from the Egyptians, that a woman who carries as an amulet or charm around her neck, the desiccated right index finger of an unborn or aborted foetus, cannot become pregnant; and likewise, in those days of constant strife and warfare with its attendant perils for women, it was customary for the ladies of noble station in life to carry with them a needle which had been dipped in dung and in the soil of a tomb, then wrapped in a piece of black cloth... for no man can have sexual congress with her as long as she carries this on her person. But then, they also knew that the same protective effect against being ravished in war was accomplished by sprinkling over the woman's body, dust from the soil upon which a mule had lain or urinated on.

And these Alchemists of old did reveal unto Princes and Potentates all manner of artifices and devises, and the means by which many truly marvellous and wonderful effects are achieved. For, the great objects of this medieval chemical science were to transmute base metals into gold, and to discover the *universal cure for diseases* and the means of indefinitely prolonging life. Thus, among other useful knowledge, they had learnt that a persistent cough is readily stopped by spitting in the mouth of that little toad that climbs trees, and allowing it to go free; and when in pain from a traumatic injury they shall spit in their hand nearest to the pain and rub the saliva unto a four footed beast, which by occultic transference receives the distress and pain. Likewise, upon passing by a dangerous or fearful place they would draw a cross with saliva on the hand and spit upon the sole of the right shoe or boot before putting it on. And no poison would be effective when a sea-star that is smeared with fox's blood is attached to a door by means of a bronze nail.

Then, Plato tells us that Gigas king of Lydia possessed a certain ring of admirable and extraordinary virtue, which when he placed it on his finger no one could see him but he could see everyone, and by it he cohabited with the Queen, killed her husband the King, slew all his opponents, and at length, by means of that ring, became King of Lydia. And as Josephus reports also of King Solomon of Jerusalem, these rings of virtues were made from the herb that is subject to a fortunate star when that star is in dominant aspect with the moon, and the images and characters of the moon are inscribed upon the congenial metal, in this case, silver.

From Plini they had learnt that there are certain toads mottled in colour and which live in the swampy mangroves; these are highly poisonous yet marvellous in their wondrous effects. For, a little bone from the *left* side of this toad when thrown in cold water will cause it to immediately boil, it will also calm vicious dogs and excite the amorous passions when taken in a potion; but the little bone that is taken from the *right* side has the opposite effect, for, when it is thrown into boiling water will instantly freeze it, and will also cure the epileptic fit when applied to the skull along with the skin of a freshly slaughtered snake, and will cool the ardour of love passions. Yet, the heart and gall bladder of these same toads are a powerful antidote against all poisons.

And so, the vast compendium of arcane, esoteric knowledge that was available to the Renaissance Alchemists was placed entirely at the disposal of the ruling Kings and Nobles of the times; but not only was the exotic art of Occult Medicine the object of their attention and investigations, for they were often called upon to act as eminent advisers to the monarchs in a wide range of state and international issues, making them especially influential and powerful in determining the outcome of the frequent intrigues and machinations that inevitably occur in the royal court and household.

As a noted Alchemist and Master Occultist, Cornelius Agrippa had fallen under the seductive temptation of the far-fetched ideals of the visionaries of his day. There was the formidable attraction that the search for the fabled 'Fountain of Youth' had on the medieval mind, and which culminated in Ponce de León's pursuit of the elusive spring in the Florida peninsula. It was the obscure writings of ancient sages that had convinced the Spanish monarchs and their advisers, of the existence of that magical fount with its potent curative waters. These were alleged to emanate from deep within the bowels of the earth, saturated with the rejuvenating virtues of elemental soil magma. It was supposed to be a suspension of precipitated primal matter in a watery vehicle, possessing the extraordinary ability of reversing the aging process and maintaining a permanent state of optimum youthfulness in all who drink *regularly* of it.

This concept of curative or 'miraculous' waters was current in a Europe that was steeped in magical lore and in various supernatural phenomena that could only be explained in terms of spiritual or divinely ordained acts. Although Ponce de León did not find the Fountain of Youth, the belief in a universal cure for diseases by means of a naturally occurring substance remained in the minds of the people, and still does.

The greatest quest, however, continued to be, especially for the Alchemist, the search for the Philosopher's Stone. And the search did continue for centuries, as the emissaries and ambassadors of the powerful European hegemonic monarchs, seeked wide and far in all known lands, for the slightest information that would throw some light or even vague insight or indication that would help in obtaining this most coveted substance or object.

Hermes, Zoroaster, Apolonius and other thaumaturgists had left the compilation of the ancient traditions in numerous writings, some of which have survived to this day. Some were written in a recognizable order, others were fragmented and disseminated in a seeming haphazard manner, but all were veiled and hidden from the superficial enquiry of the profane and the incredulous, those who are not worthy to partake of the arcane of these higher, sacred secrets. They are however, made manifest and comprehensible unto the children of wisdom and unto the diligent seekers who can discern amidst the ambiguity of apparent enigmas, that light which dispels the darkness of ignorance, common domain of the malevolent and the impious.

And Avicebron the Maurian, Avicena the Arab and Hipocrates of Cos had all left copious writings testifying to the efficacy of the Alchemical arts, and the sacred writings of these sages were well known to Agrippa and the Philosophers and Alchemists of his time. But those who seek to uncover the secret science while at the same time they are burdened by an intellectual inertia, or by the pollution of carnal commerce or by a material attachment of their sensibilities, shall not apprehend unto the truth.

The ancients all understood that there is a sort of universal soul or *primum mobile* that permeates all things through what they termed the *'quintessence'* or *fifth essence,* and that it is through this essence or 'spirit' that the occult virtues are dissemi-

19

nated unto plants, stones, metals and animals by influence of the Sun, the moon, the planets and the stars which are beyond the planets. They further explained the means by which this 'spirit' or virtue in things may be isolated and separated from its host and made useful.

Early Alchemists did seek to isolate and separate or extract this virtue from gold and to immediately apply it to a lower or baser order of metals such as lead, copper or even iron. Their success however, was limited by the fact that they could only transmute an identical weight of base metal unto gold, as that from which the virtue was extracted. This they did repeatedly, and it was accomplished in Germany, Spain, Italy and in France, as they seeked to increase the yield of transmuted gold; they failed however, in attaining unto that objective. The fact that these Alchemical experiments were conducted under the most secretive circumstances imaginable, obviated any possibility of cooperative exchange between these far-flung and widely separated artificers.

The profuse writings of Cornelius Agrippa were a vast accumulation of the combined knowledge of antiquity up to his time. In his frantic search through the records of the ancients, he had come across some provocative information of Ethiopic origins pertaining to the building of Solomon's temple in Jerusalem. The royal chronicles and traditions of that millenarian kingdom of the Nile make reference to a sacred instrument that was used in the building of the Temple, and of how this instrument was obtained through the providential actions of a rare bird, now believed to be extinct, and identified only as the "Rukh" bird[1], which is probably of the Cóndor or Eagle family.

Other corroborating data that Agrippa had previously acquired from Persian and Arabic sources, led him to seek out and obtain a specimen of the huge egg of this bird. He was intent on sub-

---

1 See in NEGUS (Majestic Tradition of Ethiopia) Chapter II for more information on the "Rukh" bird.

jecting the massive ovum to a mysterious procedure as meticulously outlined in the rare writings of the Persian sages, convinced as he was then, that he had at long last succeeded in his obsessive quest to uncover the great secret of the ages, the discovery of the fabled *'Philosopher's Stone!*

And the wisdom of the ancients holds that in the Archetypical world, that beginning source and origin of all creative ideas, words and concepts, there is One Divine Essence from whence originates all virtues and powers. As these virtues and powers are extended and disseminated through all things unto the Elemental world, it is only the *Philosopher's Stone* that is the recipient, subject and instrument of *all* natural and supernatural virtues. Thus, in it are concentrated the transmutive powers of creation in physical form that can be manipulated by mortal man for his own purposes.

Agrippa began preparations for the most exotic and demanding experiment he had ever undertaken, by having a special crucible of relatively infusible metal made. It was to be egg-shaped and capable of melting or calcining substances which require a high degree of heat over an extended period; and the size of the crucible was such that it could easily contain an average size lamb. Into it were introduced the Rukh bird's egg and equal amounts of the Alchemical elements Sulphur, Salt and Mercury, after which the crucible was firmly sealed.

The heat chamber into which it was placed seems to have been a kind of refractory oven with a contraption built in it to cause the whole crucible with its living contents to slowly and constantly rotate as heat and flames gradually act upon the metallic case, while the temperature and radiant heat do their transforming work. In fire, the mystics of old and the Alchemists saw the quintessential purifying and sacred force, which alone could bring about the changing of the vibratory nature of a material element, so that the manifestation or expression of the element is different after the change.

The ancient adept held that there is in fire an unseen virtue or 'spirit' which they called 'flogistum', and which is the transforming factor in flame and radiant heat, capable of transmuting the gross manifestations of material nature into a higher and more refined expression. They believed that in the process of that profound material change, that *transubstantiation* as it were, the 'flogistum' in fire mingles intimately with the universal essence or 'spirit' that pervades all nature, even unconscious matter, to bring about the vibratory transformation in its qualities.

Conforming to the esoteric tradition, Agrippa would maintain the crucible and egg in high heat and fire for a period of ninety days.

******

Meanwhile, the struggle for supremacy in Europe continued unabated. Charles V was the last emperor to aspire to the medieval ideal of universal empire. This Spanish and German sovereign's world-view saw the tradition of a spiritually and politically united Christian world, as the principal objective of his rulership. As king of Spain and Naples, and ruler of Milan and the Netherlands, and with an expanding colonial domain in the 'New World' of the Americas, Charles V also had the added burden of having to expel Islam from Europe and the Mediterranean. He was acutely aware of the unprecedented newness of such a task and also of the archaic nature of his antiquated administrative apparatus that would have to deal with it.

In 1522, he had to decisively quash the revolt of the *comuneros* in Spain, and even though he granted an amnesty, he also proved to be an intransigent ruler by bloodily crushing the uprising and issuing 270 death warrants. When the Turkish-Ottoman danger emerged as a clear threat to Christendom, the king was so enmeshed in the affairs of western Europe, that he had little time, energy and money left for this task. Charles V had taken advantage of his German parentage to obtain financial backing from the powerful Fugger banking family, but his finances remained in a perpetually unsettled state, as the conquests of México and Perú did not yet start to yield any significant amounts of gold for his treasury. It was not until 1550 that 17 Spanish ships provided the Emperor with some 3,000,000 ducats, in the earliest significant monetary transfusion from the New World.

It was for these reasons that Charles, already severely racked by gout, viewed Agrippa's efforts at transmuting base metals into gold, with some degree of interest, though tinged by an underlying disbelief in what he called those 'metaphysical delusions'.

In the application of fire to the concentrated repository of celestial virtues within the Rukh bird's egg, Agrippa was using the most symbolically complex phenomena in the history of human culture. Commonly found in purification rites throughout the world, fire is viewed as a powerful transformer of the negative into the positive. The Alchemical process of transmutation purifies mineral substances through pure and intense fire, then recrystallizes them in newer and higher forms. This was precisely what the old Alchemist and acknowledged expert on Occultism was fervently hoping would take place, as he patiently marked the days while keeping close watch on the crucible slowly turning in the flames that were kept alive by slaves rhythmically pressing on huge bellows.

In the considerable library of ancient manuscripts which he had accumulated in a lifetime of search and investigations, the encoded Persian descriptions of the process to obtain the fabled 'Philosopher's Stone' had seized his mind with the tenacity of an obsession. This was the most guarded secret of the ancients, one for which men had paid for with their own lives.

And, hidden within the rare Alchemical symbology was the revelation of that creative secret, always hidden from the profane and the uninitiated, which gave unto man the power to transform matter into a higher mode of its original expression.

As the time elapsed and approached sixty days since the firing of the ovum-shaped crucible, Agrippa listened keenly towards the rotating contraption. For, he had seen in one of the old parchments, a strange symbolic notation which defied a firm interpretation. It appeared to him that the meaning was 'Unto sixty days, the unborn bird levitates'. So he listened attentively, revealing to none other what he inclined to hear... then he realized that the rumbling sound of the egg as it rolled within its metallic enclosure, was gone. He approached the kiln-oven as close he could because of the intense heat, then he became convinced that indeed it was true, that after sixty days the Rukh bird's egg would seemingly float, that is, levitate, and remain suspended in mid-space within the crucible for the next thirty days.

It had shrunk to less than one third its original size, and was now entering into the stage of recrystallization. Every other preparation had already been made. There was fourteen tons of lead stacked nearby along with a small amount of "seed" gold on it, and a huge double-thong capable of lifting the ovum from the crucible while it is still at its extreme temperature.

The entire chamber where the alchemical procedure was taking place, radiated with an unusual heat which proceeded from the fiery kiln. The constant and steady flames were fueled by a rare mixture of bituminous coal, anthracite and lignite (brown coal) along with a proportionate amount of the stone *asbestos* which, once lit, remains burning for an extremely long period of time, with an intensity that is surprising for its concentrated flame and elevated heat emissions.

At exactly ninety days since the start of Agrippa's alchemical experiment, the crucible was opened, revealing its transformed contents which was no longer the original large egg of the Rukh bird, but rather an extremely luminous and incandescent blue sphere, the brightness of which filled the chamber and bathed all in its incredibly intense luminosity and penetrating radiant heat.

Under the Alchemist's methodical directions, the spherical 'Philosopher's Stone' was grasped with the thongs and moved towards the stack of lead nearby, where it was carefully placed upon the small block of 'seed' gold that was exactly on the top and center of the large pile of compacted lead. Agrippa had ensured that the gold to be used was of the 'expanded' type and not of the 'contracted' form, and would therefore be able to transubstantiate a quantum of base metal many times its own weight.

As the 'Stone' touched the square of gold, a burst of gaseous vapour came forth and it appeared as if the intensely glittering and brilliant blue stone was absorbing the gold unto itself without melting any of it, and so, there was no metal liquefaction at all. Slowly, over a period of twenty days, the stone which had then absorbed all of the gold, descended with its searing heat through the entire stockpile of lead, and as it passed through, the lead would be gradually transmuted into pure gold. But at the end of the process, it was found that the 'Philosopher's Stone' had been dissipated through the metal and that none of it remained.

Chapter 3

The Arcanum
of Occult Medicine

For King Charles V, the success of Agrippa's alchemy meant a change of fortunes and a significant alteration in the direction of the kingdom's extensive international spread. Spain was involved in serious disputes with France, with the Turks under Suleyman the Magnificent and even with the Papacy under Pope Clement VII. Charles was also intent on conquering North Africa, but his attention was sorely needed elsewhere, as his domains in North Germany were on the brink of revolt.

Under the severe pressures brought about by a series of military and diplomatic setbacks, as well as his deteriorating health, Charles abdicated the throne in favour of his son Philip II under whose reign Spain would achieve its greatest power and widest geographical extent. Philip had become increasingly concerned at the growing support that both England and France were giving to the rebellious provinces of the Netherlands, and eventually became convinced that the Catholic religion in Western Europe, and his own authority in the Netherlands, could only be saved by open intervention against England and France.

To that end he began outfitting the *Armada* which, with the help of the Spanish army in the Netherlands was intended to conquer England in 1588. It was the inherited wealth coming partially from the alchemical transmutation of base metal into gold that was achieved during his father's reign, that allowed Philip to embark on that enterprise by which he hoped to crush Britain's imperial world hegemony.

Originally estimated to number 556 ships carrying 94,000 men, this staggering force nevertheless suffered an epoch-making defeat, which saved England and the Protestant Reformation as well. As history would have it, not even the Alchemist's gold could prevail against mighty Britannia, she who was prophetically destined to 'rule the waves' and establish an empire over which 'the sun never sets'.

And although these Alchemists of old many times functioned as physicians in the King's courts, they also proffered advice pertaining to a wide variety of situations as well as the means of achieving desired effects for virtually any condition faced then.

And in the writings of Cornelius Agrippa, he makes reference to the well-known virtue of magnets which attracts iron, yet, as soon as a diamond is brought close to it this virtue disappears because diamonds are of opposing virtue to all magnets. Thus, they practiced the arcane art of Occult Medicine, of which one of the Sages, Pselle the Plantonic, recommended carrying on the person the head, heart or eyes of crows, roosters or bats for boldness in any endeavours; and in like manner, it is stated that a crow's heart or the head of a bat will surely keep whoever carries it, fully awake, when it is tied on to the right arm.

During those days of fourteenth century medieval Europe, these exotic remedies and artifices were quite frequently resorted to, and formed part of the deeply ingrained beliefs and practices of the people; all these eventually evolved over time to coalesce into a strange amalgam of ritual, magic, science and superstition.

Yet, the Alchemical art of the adept remained a fairly precise body of ancient knowledge with specified procedures and methods, which they took pains to conceal under the seeming enigma of their encoded writings.

Thus they state that some rabbit fat or the heart of an owl when placed over the left breast of a sleeping woman, will cause her to reveal all manner of secret things without awaking; and a woman who each month drinks one measure of her cupped hand of the urine of a mule will not be impregnated. Their copious arcane writings make reference to the virtues inherent in any of a number of serpents and snakes which renew and rejuvenate their bodies by the periodic shedding of their skins; and to this day in the Orient, traditional Chinese medicine prescribes the eating of serpents to achieve an overall rejuvenation of tired and fatigued bodies.

There is a herb known as 'bee's rice' which is much coveted by serpents and all reptiles, and when eaten by man, ensures that one dies 'laughing'. Yet, when a stork or an ibis is stung by a serpent, it is cured by eating the herb *Oregano;* and it is known that the *Oregano* has strong virtues against poisons. In like manner for all forms of melancholic, depressive and nervous conditions, they achieved a wonderful cure with the herb known as *Adianta* or 'Hair of Venus'.

In the frequent wars and minor skirmishes so common in his day, it was through the writings of Agrippa that the herb *dictamme* came to be used for arrow wounds, for when wounded men eat of it, all embedded arrows and darts are forthwith repelled and ejected from the body. He further recorded the efficacy of applying a freshly killed rat to a scorpion sting, noting the almost immediate reduction of pain and swelling. And these phenomena confirm the interconnectedness of the entire creation and the interplay of diffused virtues at all levels of the animal, mineral and plant domains, at times relating to each other in harmony, but at other times are found in antagonic opposition.

So it was observed from antiquity that serpents and crabs are contrary to each other, and that swines stung by serpents cure themselves by eating crabs. That enmity and opposition even extends to the celestial realm, for, when the sun is in the sign of Cancer, serpents remain constantly encoiled; and if a crocodile is merely touched with a feather of the Egyptian sunbird, which feeds on serpents, he is instantly paralyzed. From ancient historian Orus Apollon they had learnt that one who wears the skin of a hyena, may easily pass through the ranks of an enemy camp with impunity and boldness. But opposite, antagonic virtues are also noted when a promiscuous woman plants an olive tree; it becomes either sterile, or the tree itself becomes permanently dried up.

And the lion fears nothing more than lit torches, and he cannot be tamed but by means of fire; likewise, the wolf fears not the lance, arrow or iron, only the stone which inflicts upon him a sore that becomes festered with maggots. They knew also of the effectual curse upon snakes, for, when a nude man with extended arms and legs faces a serpent it is instantly immobilized, yet will attack him when he is dressed.

The ancient Alchemists did realize that there are those virtues which are diffused through the whole body of the animal or plant, as there are other instances where the peculiar virtue or power is concentrated in only one part of the body or in one organ. The *Echeneis* or Remora, can easily stop the movement of a ship or of another big fish, with the virtue that pervades its entire body. And this little fish has a suctorial disk on the head with which he clings to other fishes or to ships. Thus they also found that the hyena has throughout its whole body that virtue by which, if dogs come even near to its shadow, they are unable to bark.

The Arcane Science postulates that the stronger virtues and powers are those that reside in only one part, organ or appendage of the animal or plant, like in the eyes only, or the tongue or some other part; and so it is known that there is a very violent virtue in the eyes of the *Basilisk,* for, it will cause men to die instantly if one looks into its eyes. And this *Basilisk* is a fabulous serpent, lizard or a kind of dragon whose breath and looks are fatal. They usually have a membranous bag on the head that can be filled with air, and an erectile crest along the back. They noted also a similar virtue in the eyes of the hyena, as her gaze upon any animal stunts and immobilizes it. The wizards had concocted certain *Coliriums* or eye-slaves made from the eyes of selected animals, to bring about similar effects and fascinations or enchantments.

Paracelsus, the noted Swiss Occult Physician, had observed in his writings that poultry fed on fox's liver, are avoided by foxes and other rodents, which pointed to the induced diffusion of natural virtues merely by eating a certain organ or part of an animal. Paracelsus spoke also of the many ways in which diverse virtues are expanded through certain body parts, thus, the eyes receive from on high the virtue of sight, ears the virtue of hearing, but it is the bones which receive in concentrated form the vital life force or the negative polarity of matter. He made reference to a very small, round and smooth bone in the human body, apparently non-functional, of about the size of a green pea, and which the Hebrews call *Luz;* it cannot be broken or burnt with fire, and if it remains whole, from it will emerge our earthly body at the resurrection of the dead, like a plant from its seed.

In those plants exhibiting a *tropism* in which sunlight is the orienting stimulus, such as the heliotropes, which turns or bends towards the sun, the concentrated virtues it has upon the sun's rays are truly admirable, for, it turns them into blood, that is, it makes the sun appear as in eclipse, once it is rubbed with the herb of its same name, heliotrope, and placed in a glass full of water. It also has another marvellous virtue upon men's eyes, which is to annul their function, sharpness and penetrative power, to the extent that it prevents others from seeing anyone who carries on his person both plant and herb tied together. This was also confirmed by Albertus Magnus and Aesculapius in the book of his epistles to Octavius Augustus.

They had mentioned also the rare stone *Pyrophilos* which is of a red mottled colour and has an admirable virtue against all manner of poisons. It was called *Evanthum* by Aaron the High Priest. It is a solar stone and it will turn glorious and formidable before his enemies, anyone who carries it on his person.

From the Zoroastrians they had learnt the art of invisible writings, and of how the heat from fire will make visible that which was written with milk or the juice of onions. Out in the fields the spies left markings on the rocks with goat's fat which are totally invisible until they are bathed in vinegar; then they will appear as if sculpted upon the stone, revealing the movement of enemy troops.

And many other wonderful effects were made manifest by the appropriate admixture of plants, flowers, animal parts and organs, or certain mineral substances or stones which they concocted in various unguent, coliriums and potions, as it has been abundantly recorded by Arquitas, Democritus and Hermes in his book called Alchorat, in the books of Quirámides and in the works of many other ancient Philosophers, Alchemists and Historians. For, all the Magical Arts and all the Secret Philosophy confirms that there is such a connection and continuity in nature and that the Celestial virtues through the expansion of its rays, affects continuously and concomitantly everything in the earthly realm. And there is nothing that escapes this influence, nor is there any material substance that is not susceptible to these virtues.

Although the operations of celestial virtues would manifest in certain marvellous ways, many times these natural effects and their mechanism were incomprehensible to the ancients. So, in the Book of Nemith, also known as 'The Laws of Pluto' reference is made to the grotesque or monstrous creations that are not according to the laws of nature. And there it is stated that a crab buried without its claws and feet will generate scorpions; that the duck that is burnt to ashes and thrown into the water will generate toads; and the hairs of a menstruating woman, when placed under a pile of straw will bring forth serpents. Likewise, the introduction of the seed of an ass into the mare, which brings forth the barren mule, was the signal creation of the Gomorraites, and was not ordained by nature.

And they comprehended not the actuating effect of virtues which caused that little fish called *Echeneis* or Remora, if its body is cut in sections and thrown into the sea, that these will readily unite and the fish revives. Or that which is concentrated in the ball of the hyena's eyes, since when placed under the tongue will give the faculty of divination, and the same effect will be obtained with the lunar stone, *Selenite.*

The admirable virtue of certain poisons are referred to in the writings of Miguel Scoto, and he instructs those who would learn, that the stomach of an antelope when burnt to ashes and mixed with the menstrual blood of a woman as in a piece of cloth, whoever carries this on his person will be immune from arrows, lance and any projectile. And the menstrual blood of women has such powerful virtues in it, that it will annual the power of any enchantment when it is applied to the doorposts of a house; if it goes upon a vine, will at once render it sterile; it will kill trees and dry their fruit; makes the sharp edge of knives and swords dull, and will immediately rust iron tools.

In the writings of Severino Boecio mention is made of the metal by which a man has been killed; if spurs and bit are made of it and the sign of the intelligence of Mercury are inscribed on them, it is then possible to tame and ride the friskiest horse. And if horseshoes are made of that fatal metal with the same inscriptions carved on them, the horse shod with them becomes extremely swift and tireless. And the cure for the *Grand Mal,* a strongly marked form of epilepsy, is had by obtaining the metal that had killed a man, and placing it in a cup of port wine which is put outside under the full moon for three consecutive nights. When this is drunk by the sick person he will be permanently cured.

Boecio also discloses that if someone buries or hides gold, silver or any other valuable thing, then fumigates the place with a mixture of equal parts of coriander, saffron and black sleeping grass, no one will be able to find or to remove the hidden object, for they would be under the custody of demons, who will cause any but the person that placed it there, to be tormented and maddened if he attempts to remove it. Only burning sulphur will obliterate the powerful enchantment and demonic protection therein.

According to Plini, quoting from the arcane writings of Anaxilao, if the coital fluid of mares is taken and burnt or heated, monstrous forms and heads of horses will appear, and the same happens with asses. Likewise, the skin of a serpent when burnt with fire will bring forth serpents. And so, as they were adept at manipulating fire and light in various forms, they were also aware of the hidden force of enchantments and visual rays. Thus, the most passionate of love affairs are lit with a single look through the power of the rays emanating from the eyes, and which like an arrow strikes through the eyes of the recipient and is expanded throughout the whole body and all its members.

In the vast compendium of rare and exotic remedies available to the Occult practitioner of Medieval Europe, truly incomprehensible and baffling procedures are found. Plini again, mentions that an undulating fever is cured by dropping nail clippings from the patient on an ants nest, then taking the ant that picked up the first clipping and after killing it, placing it on the neck of the affected person, bringing about an immediate cure. By mixing the nail clippings with candle-wax a swift remedy is also obtained; but if a piece of wood burnt by a ray of lightning is flung behind with his hands by a sick person, he is instantly cured of any ailment affecting him.

Plini again states that if an iron nail is placed under the pillow where an epileptic rests his head, it will be an effective remedy against this malady after it is put into a cup of port wine that is allowed to absorb the full moon's rays for three consecutive nights; it is then drunk by the patient. He also records the well known custom of taking any herb or twigs that may appear upon the head of a statue, which, when tied unto any part of one's garments will immediately cure a headache. And an effective remedy against migraine headache is obtained by only once bathing the head with an infusion of the plant 'Purple Jew'.

The ancient practitioner of Occult Medicine recognized the formal qualities of *light* upon all things and all living beings, which are affected by the virtues of light according to their individual capacities. Thus it is, that the Sages did not permit the shadow of an ill person to fall upon anything, nor for their urine to be exposed to sunlight or moonlight, for their penetrating rays would actuate the noxious elements, contaminating the healthy by action of the 'vapours' that would be disseminated in the immediate area. They always ensured then, that it would be the shadow of the physician that would cover the patient and not otherwise.

Numerous other observations of the ancients which bring forth marvellous effects, further illustrates the pervasiveness of the subtle links that exists throughout all creation, by reason of the dissemination of celestial virtues. And so, they would alleviate the pains of childbirth by placing on the bed a stone, arrow or iron which has killed either a man, a wildhog or a bear. They noticed also that an arrow extracted from a body, without touching the ground, when placed in the bed will generate intense amorous passions.

When planted fields are threatened by intense storms and high winds, at that very time, a rooster would be caught and split between two men who would separately circumambulate the field in opposing directions, and after meeting at the starting point would there bury the two halves. This method they found to be highly effective in protecting the fields from devastation by the high winds. And it was Albertus Magnus quoting Chiránides who informs us that in order to annual the love-enchantment of a woman, one needs only to urinate on the right hand sleeve of her blouse; this will destroy the spell.

Albertus also expounded on the poison that resides in the knees of a pregnant woman, and thus advises against remaining in close contact with one or both knees; and in the councils of Dukes, Princes and Potentates it was forbidden for anyone to cross legs by placing one upon the knee, for it was deemed to prevent any useful decisions or action. They also claimed that if a man who is lying with a woman inside a house is called by his name and when he answers, a needle or a knife with broken point is attached to the door outside, that man will not be able to perform the 'labours of Venus' as long as the needle or the knife remains attached to the door.

Among the ancients, the art or practice of augury or divination by means of omens, and through the observation and interpretation of the actions and movements of animals and of natural phenomena, was a well established one and frequently consulted by kings and nobles. For it was widely believed that in all things there are hidden oracles which predict coming events, and this is so especially in the birds of omen or of prognostication whom they claimed were the reincarnated souls of men, returned as birds. And so, Epictetus, the Stoic Philosopher and author, stated that when a crow screeches upon seeing someone, it is prognosticating negative things about his health, his honour or fortunes, his wife and children. The Eagle is considered the most reliable bird of omen, as it soars far above all other birds, its sight is more profound and penetrating, and it prognosticates exaltation and victory, but only by means of blood, for it drinks not water but only blood.

Historically it is known that an eagle which suddenly perched upon Hieron's shield, while he was conducting his first campaign, predicted that he would be king. And the two eagles that remained all day long on the roof of the house where Alexander of Macedonia (the Great) was born, predicted that he would be master of two empires, Asia and Europe. When Lucio Tarquino, son of Demaratho of Corinth, fled his country because of a sedition, he went first to Etruria and then left towards Rome; an eagle clasped his hat and flew high with it, prognosticating that he would be king of the Romans.

Crows on the other hand, portend difficulties, tribulations and cruelty by reason of rapine or pillage. Whenever these birds remain for up to seven days facing the field where a battle is to be fought, they always look towards that area where the defeated army will be, as if anticipating the feast of slaughtered bodies that awaits them. They invariably signal the defeat of an army. For that reason the monarchs of old would send people to observe where the crows were perched and in what direction they were looking. According to Almaden, when two hawks, or two birds of the same kind fight each other, it signifies revolution within a kingdom.

When a rat-bat encounters someone who is fleeing, it is considered a good omen for the fleeing person, for although the bat has no wings, he does not cease to fly. The turtledove is bad omen for he who flees, but is a good sign for lovers for when in heat will copulate with the female seven times each hour. Bees are a powerful prognostication for kings and rulers; it signifies the obedience of nations. House flies indicate troublesome molestation and embarrassment, for though they be chased away, always return. Livia, the mother of Tiberius, when she was pregnant with this child, kept in her bosom a chicken's egg until it hatched a rooster with large crest; the sages interpreted this to mean that the child to be born would be king. Likewise a beaver, which when pursued will leave the hunter his testicles which he has torn off with his own teeth, is a bad augury and means that a man will do great harm to himself.

Signs and portents were also noted at the birth or infancy of great and notable men, as Cicero states about King Midas in whose mouth while asleep, ants placed grains of wheat forecasting great wealth for him; likewise the bees which perched upon young Plato's mouth while he was asleep, predicted for him the gift of eloquence.

Josephus, in his History of Jerusalem, tells us of a mysterious plant known as *Root of Baaras* and which grows near the Judean town of *Macherunte*. It is the colour of fire and gives off a bright luminosity, yet is difficult of grasping for it somehow eludes hands and sight, and will only remain still after sprinkling with urine from a menstruating woman. It is still dangerous even after immobilizing it this way, for, if pulled from the ground will cause the immediate death of whomever plucked it unless he is protected by an amulet previously made with that kind of root. The sages would dig around the root and tie a cord around it which is attached to a dog who pulls at it in order to follow his master, and so, finally tears the root from the earth and dies instantly. Thereafter it can be handled safely. This root has extremely powerful virtues for casting evil spirits out of possessed bodies, as its mere proximity to the tormented person will attract the evil entity, expelling it out of the body it occupies, usually through the nostrils actuated by a sneeze.

The primitive church, and right up to the renaissance era, did use certain types of enchantments and Occult methods and procedures against a variety of illnesses, and would have maintained a virtual monopoly on the traditional healing arts were it not for the emerging relevance and practical efficiency of the Alchemical and Scientific discoveries and their application.

The Cosmology or 'Worldview' of the Alchemist was one that was far beyond that of the Medieval mind of their era. Its sophistication and analytical complexity was partly due to the accumulated wisdom of the ancients, a tradition of mystery and awesomeness surrounding the carefully nurtured secrets of the universe, of creation, the nature of man and his ultimate destiny. Around this body of revealed knowledge the ancient philosophical brotherhoods and mystery schools grew in many lands. The Knight Templars, The Freemasons of the Scottish Rite, the Rosicrucians and others, made up this exclusive elite of privileged possessors of a secret knowledge, an arcane gnosis which they zealously guarded lest it fall into the hands of the profane.

They had journeyed long and persistently through the mystical path of spiritual search which had prepared them to receive the sacred oracles. For, after imbibing in the mundance teachings of empirical sciences, their admittance into the Mystery school as Neophytes, sealed their destiny, because they had begun that irreversible transition from the realms of darkness into that of light, and from the slavery of falsehood into the truth that liberates.

Then, it was as a Postulant to the higher degrees of the Metaphysical studies in the centuries-old Philosophical schools, that the embryonic Alchemist was deemed to be sufficiently prepared to receive the transcendental truths known only to a small, select circle of adepts. The various stages and degrees they went through was punctuated by a set of rituals and ceremonies of initiation which prepares the Postulant for the next stage or degree.

This mystery of initiation is revealed to the Neophyte entering the First Atrium of the Higher Studies of the Order, through a ceremony which he performs privately or in the Temple, and where the classic geometric figures of Circle and Triangle are used along with candles and incense, in a ritual which prepares the Subconscious Mind to grasp and fully comprehend the profound concepts and truths known to the Sages of remote antiquity.

The initiatory rite is also a test or a trial of the Postulant, as his resolve, determination, and above all, courage, are balanced and must not be found wanting. For, entering the Higher Studies he will know and understand that "Deity resides only within Man"; that Time and Space have no existence in reality, but are illusions of the mortal mind of man, conceived by man in his need to understand the world and assign order and sequence to observable events.

Later on, as he advances through the various stages of his continuous preparation, another initiatory ritual requires the use of a human skull, which must be from one who has died violently in his prime, and preferably one who was homicidal, for, the negative polarity of the spirit force in man would be highly concentrated in such skull, making it easier to be invoked and manipulated through the use of fire, rum and 'Dragon's Blood' or 'Blood of Saturn'. It is for this reason principally, that executed manslayers are not interred in public cemeteries or 'holy ground' as they would be dug out swiftly by necromancers and others seeking the skull.

And it was precisely for one of these advanced initiatory ceremonies, that, many years ago in another land, I had gone to a remote Indian burial ground in search of an appropriate skull. Young and recklessly bold, I had cajoled a neighbour's gardener, Joselo, to come and do the exhumation, for which he was promised a good monetary reward. We arrived at the grave around the ninth hour that night and Joselo started digging rapidly while I kept watch. I had been told that these Indian cemeteries are always guarded by spirits; this I did not mention to my assistant, but I came prepared for any challenge from that realm.

I was greatly amazed to discover after much digging, that the body was contained in a kind of crude stone coffin, a true sarcophagus, since the stone used was a type of limestone which has the effect of disintegrating within a few weeks the flesh of the bodies deposited in it. The box was also brittle, and with one strike of the shovel it cracked like pumice. I quickly pushed my hand through the gaping cavity but felt only pieces of bone and stone fragments and dust from the coffin; I realized then that this was the lower extremity and that the head would be at the other end.

Both of us were in the hole and actually standing on parts of the fragmenting coffin, and as I struck the other end with the shovel breaking up that part of the box, a shrieking, howling sound which seemed to surround us, instantly paralyzed us. I turned swiftly only to see Joselo literally leap out of the hole seemingly with wings on his feet. I dropped to a crouch and felt with my hands the round and surprisingly lightweight bony ball of the desiccated cranium, while at the same time shouting for Joselo to come back.

The horrendous blood-curdling sound seemed to get louder as I wrapped the skull in the black cloth I had, and placed it in my shoulder bag. I then rapidly sprinkled some of the rum I carried in a flask, palmed my ceremonial dagger from its sheath and climbed out of the hole. I ran in the direction we had come, and as I approached a small stream near to the winding village dirt track, the howling scream that had been following me got closer and louder. I knelt on a little sand-clearing by the stream's edge and quickly drew a cross in the sand with the dagger which I then stuck in the center of the cross, then I plucked a strand of hair from my head and placed it under my tongue; at this, the chilling scream ceased. As for the gardener Joselo, he positively avoided me at all costs, and he even refused to accept an envelope with the promised money that I sent him.

The skull was a well-developed mature one of about thirty eight years at time of death, and had no evident traumatic injuries to it. A typical orthognatous skull, that is, one in which the angle made by the intersection of the axis of the face with the axis of the skull is around ninety degrees, made it round rather than elongated, and the highly developed supraorbital ridges it had gave it a kind of fixed, concentrated gaze.

It did not, however, remain long in my possession, for, shortly after fulfilling its ritualistic purposes, was found to be missing from the hiding place designated for its safekeeping. This was really baffling since I had to rule out theft or trickery; it just disappeared and no reasonable explanation for this was ever arrived at. The initiatory process along with the trials one undergoes to obtain all that is required for the ceremony, both prove to be stringent tests not only formulated to determine one's resolve and unshakable will, but also to instill in the consciousness a fearlessness and boldness of spirit that will enable one to face virtually any situation armed with the rare knowledge of the ancients.

That intimately subjective experience empowers the Adept with a kind of inner fire, a discerning light, while the symbolism used in the initiatory ritual conveys in a particularly dramatic manner, certain timeless concepts and ideas through the awakening of the subconscious mind, and by evoking memories and experiences of past lives. For, the doctrine of reincarnation which holds that the soul transmigrates through a series of lives in cycles of birth, death and rebirth was fully understood by the Alchemists and Philosophers of old.

These initiatory mysteries have lived on through the ages with their rituals and mystical exercises transmitted from generation to generation; from its recorded beginnings at around 1350 BC in ancient Egypt under the Pharaoh Akhnaton, through many cycles and periods of centuries-long dormancy, unto its emergence in the Middle Ages with the Knight Templars' prominence during the Crusades to liberate Jerusalem from Islamic rule.

To the Alchemist and the Occult Physician, remedial medicine did not heal but rather suppressed, neutralized or banished symptoms, and it was Consciousness which originated every imbalance that manifests in the body. And although symptoms can help in finding the cause of various pathologies, symptomatic relief only puts off acceptance of the lessons that symptoms give. Bodies do not just get sick nor does disease travel from person to person, neither do germs spread disease, since disease organisms are always present and arise when the body is making an attempt to clear imbalance it can no longer hold. Disease organisms are actually a part of the body that is always ready to clear itself of any invasion that is life-threatening.

They regarded the human body as that perfect harmonic expression of the universe, the "Microcosm", carrying in the proportion of its measurements and the symmetry of all its parts, the Divine universal code of perfect creation. Thus the ancients designed and erected their buildings, temples, columns and pedestals, homes and palaces according to the measurements and proportions of the human body. Thus, the height, width, depth and circumference of the human body correspond in proportion to the measurements of the heavenly bodies.

They conceived the four fluids in man to be in perfect arithmetic proportion, determining a person's health and temperament. These four fluids or humours are blood, phlegm, choler (yellow bile) and melancholy (black bile) and in the normal man there are eight portions of blood, four of phlegm, two of choler, and one of melancholy. These fluids are subject to the gravitational pull of the moon and to a lesser extent to that of the other heavenly bodies, and this has been observed with cranial blood and menstrual blood, and it is known that if the full moon's light-rays should rest upon a person's face while sleeping, it can bring about facial rictus, palsy or partial paralysis of the facial muscles. Thus the importance they ascribed to the effects of celestial influences on the entire creation.

Classical anatomists had discovered certain nerve around the neck, which, when stimulated will cause the movement of every limb and member of the body according to its natural movement. Aristoteles claimed that God with a similar stimulation gives movement to all the parts of creation. They further described the two branches of a vein also around the throat, which, if pressured sharply at the point where they divide near the throat, will cause immediate loss of consciousness until released.

Mystics and Metaphysicians long ago recognized certain influences and powers of a cosmic nature which permeates all of creation. The endocrine or ductless glands which control a range of physical and mental functions, are the medium in our bodies for the reception of this 'Divine Energy'. They act as governors or 'transformers' of this cosmic energy, and can either speed up or slow down its influx into the body.

Of the endocrine glands, the pineal and the pituitary in their physiological purpose, have to do with the regulating of such functions of the body such as the circulation of the blood, the growth of the bones and tissues, and the development of the sexual and emotional functions. But in the psychic sense, they are really like transformers, stepping down for objective sensing those exceedingly rapid vibrations from the spiritual or psychic planes, so that they may be sensed on the material plane. Thus, these ancient mystics were aware of the pineal gland as the most efficient transformer of the Cosmic energy into rates of vibrations which are discernible by our objective minds, a true Third Eye appearing as an appendage of the brain present in all craniate vertebrates. Though little understood by mundane sciences, it is evidently the remnant of an important sense organ in ancestral form. They knew that by a series of mystical exercises, this gland may be stimulated and brought to its peak performance, which through a process of a seeming Divine Alchemy can readily restore an organism to its original perfection in harmony with the macrocosm or universe.

Although the Medieval Church condemned the dissection of human bodies, it is obvious from historical records that the practice was clandestinely widespread throughout most of Europe; and so, the master of Occult Medicine had ample opportunity to conduct detailed and exhaustive observation of morbid pathologies or diseased organs, tissue, glands and viscera in cadavers.

The voluminous notes contained in Agrippa's published works and in his unpublished private papers, reveal a surprisingly comprehensive and profound knowledge of most illnesses. And it was through the painful process of empirical trial and error along with the revealed gnosis of the mystics, that a formidable Pharmacology of natural, crude and simple remedies and cures was accumulated. To this they added of course, the plethora of exotic, arcane Occult methods, many of which were of a purely Meta-physical, Spiritistic or Alchemical nature.

Cornelius Agrippa had outraged Charles V with the publication in 1530 of a scathing attack on Occultism and all sciences in his work *"On the Vanity and Uncertainty of Sciences"*. The King had been suffering for some time from Acute Gouty Arthritis caused mainly by his overindulgence in food and alcohol. This condition became chronic with the typical progressively excruciating pain at the metatarsophalangeal joint of the big toe, which had become swollen and exquisitely tender, due to effusion into the joint space and edema of the surrounding soft tissues.

But, another clinical entity was associated with the king's chronic gout, possibly leukemia, a form of cancer of the blood-forming tissues, in which the increased formation of purine substances may also lead to uric acid deposits in joints and acute articulate attacks, usually of nocturnal onset, just as in gout.

When Agrippa told the king that other, more life-threatening processes which would require radical modes of treatment were the underlying causes of his painful condition, he refused to believe that his ailment was anything other than gout. King Charles V disposition towards Agrippa had changed and became one of almost open hostility, as the king believed that Agrippa's controversial work against all sciences would inevitably stimulate the Renaissance revival of Skepticism, which he perceived as being another form of mental aberration threatening the powers of both, Church and State.

Agrippa's exacting and uncompromising traits, along with his refusal to recant the denunciation and rejection of all Arts and Sciences, forced him to leave the Spanish court to take refuge under the French Burgundian monarchs. Well received at first, he became personal physician to Louise of Savoy, and it was during this period that he accomplished some of his most dramatic and impressive cures. In those days the many instances of "Grand Mal' (Falling Sickness, Epilepsy), constituted a truly frightening and mysterious endemic illness of unknown origin and ethiology.

This paroxysmal disorder of cerebral function, manifests as convulsive seizure attacks which are sudden in onset and of short duration, with changes in the state of consciousness. Agrippa, and other Occult Physicians in Medieval Europe had recognized that Epileptic seizures were many times caused by spiritistic activity, where the subject's spectrum of visual vibrations is briefly expanded through neuronal stimulation of sight centers in the brain. Consequently, the patient at times sees non-material beings, commonly called *"Fallen Angels",* the sight of which brings about paroxysmal episodes marked by convulsions and loss of consciousness due to the sudden alteration of the individual's magnetic aura.

This disruption of the person's aural integrity is caused by the proximity to a being of a higher vibratory level, and is electrical in nature. The higher vibratory frequency creates a form of electromagnetic storm throughout the nervous system, manifesting as the convulsions of an epileptic seizure. This malady, which is still little understood by mundane science was successfully treated by Agrippa, as documented in his private papers and corroborated by other Thaumaturgists and Occultists in their writings.

To the medieval man and woman of that era, the rare, exotic and mysterious methods used by the Alchemist and the Occult Physician in the treatment of various illnesses and cases of demonic possession and evil enchantments, were not considered weird or unorthodox procedures, but rather the normal, standard practices of the Alchemical artificer. For in those days, the perennial and constant preoccupation of all and sundry, was the iniquitous ministry of evil carried out by the demoniacal host of the 'Prince of Darkness'.

Thus, women were visited at night by the *Incubus,* a nightmarish evil spirit of insatiable venereal appetite and lasciviousness, which would have sexual intercourse with sleeping women, forcing them to engage in depraved, abnormal forms of sexual congress and committing with them all manner of unspeakable abominations. The victims were subsequently treated by ingesting a concoction made with the fleshy pulp of the hard-shelled bottle-gourd (Calabash), a powerful abortifacient which seemed to restore the demon-ravished dame to some semblance of normality.

Males in turn, would in their sleep be drained of their seminal fluid by the *Succubus,* a demon assuming female form and exhibiting intense Nymphomania (or uterine fire, insatiable sexual appetite), which would subject them to prolonged and exhausting coitus. A sequela to the erotic, nocturnal encounter, is a chronic drip of ejaculatory fluid, which the Occult Physician cured instantly by having the patient leap three times over an open flame.

It is known that the ordinary people of Persia (Iran, today) used vaccination long before Dr. Jenner of England noticed the cowpox on the hands of a dairymaid. In Elizabethan England, the use of *Foxglove* for edema or dropsy was practiced by a so-called Shropshire witch. She gathered herbs by the light of the full moon, when the lunar gravitational pull would draw the sap towards leaves and branches, and making a concoction of them, successfully treated Queen Elizabeth. Only much later was it learned that the effective herb of all the plants she used was *Foxglove* or *Digitalis,* which is effectively used to this day in the treatment of heart failure and its accompanying edema.

The superstitious medieval man lived in constant fear of illnesses, those insidious, silent and treacherous processes in his own body which to his mind were 'spirit-mediated'. The widespread ravages of the fourteenth century plague epidemic, the 'Black Death', which wiped out fully one-third of Europe's population, had left a permanent impression upon his mind and that of generations to come.

Abnormalities still evident in ancient skeletons bear mute witness of bone infections, arthritis, tumours, and the unexplained disappearance of entire tribes and clans, and the discovery of burial grounds filled with youthful bodies, suggest the havoc wrought by epidemics. Ancient records carry many references to *Pestilentia,* the epidemics of highly communicable infecto-contagious diseases for which no cause was known.

That condition anciently described as 'a crablike monster gnawing at the entrails', 'the wasting disease that rests not unto the grave' and many other quaintly descriptive terms, undoubtedly refers to the same terminal illness seen in three-thousand year old mummies of ancient Egypt, *Cancer.* And in the ancient world, Egypt's physicians commanded great respect for their knowledge of anatomy and surgery; however, learning in specialized fields was a secret endeavour, and this secrecy of learning seems to have been general. This was true of medicine, and even writing, the art of the scribes, was a secret science. And it was from ancient Egypt that Europe had received a formidable corpus of medical knowledge which greatly augmented the already wide spectrum of skills at the disposal of their physicians. During its 3,000 years of recorded history (3100 BC – 50 BC) Egypt was ruled by at least 350 Pharaohs through thirty dynasties. Between 1600 and 1000 BC Egyptian dentists were restoring teeth with bridges. Mineral drugs were used, among them one that cannot be identified today and which produced anesthesia so as to make surgical operations possible without suffering.

The Egyptian physician knew about the arteries and how to count the pulse; they knew the relationship of the heart to the lungs and how to treat fractures and set bones. They also had knowledge of sutures and cauterizing, and used scalpels, scissors and forceps. *The Ebers Medical Papyrus* and *The Edwin Smith Surgical Papyrus,* the latter derived from sources dating to the time of the Old Kingdom (2700 BC – 2200 BC), lists an enormous number of prescriptions for countless herbs, draughts, fomentations, ointments, coliriums and liniments for a wide variety of illnesses.

The functions of the heart are given great attention in both manuscripts, displaying a recognition of the organic relation of the heart to the various parts of the body, and that the heart may be the source of life. *The Ebers Papyrus* deals largely with the heart, and it states there that: "There are vessels in it which go to every part of the body". *The Smith Papyrus* deals largely with broken bones, and describes some 48 cases including fractures of ribs, clavicle, skull and dislocations of the jaw.

Much of the millenarian Egyptian medical arts was added to the European, Celtic, Gothic tradition during Rome's three centuries of world empire, which encompassed Egypt and most of North Africa. The ancient Egyptian physician had an extensive range of prescriptions they used for such afflictions as respiratory distress, gastric and digestive disorders, hemorrhages, constipation; for the latter they prescribed castor oil. Dental problems and disorders of the gum, headaches and eye troubles were all treated routinely, and extensive use was made of linen for bandages, medical dressings, and large quantities for the wrapping of mummies.

It still baffles the mind whenever we contemplate the level of sophistication, the consummate skill and wide knowledge that was achieved by the Masters of Medicine under the Pharaohs of Egypt. For they had the means of treating tumours, abscesses and hernia, and had an understanding of the relationship between the nervous system and the voluntary movements of the body. They were also able to localize a condition of paralysis, depending on the situation of a nerve lesion. But then, consistent with the exclusivist perspective of all ancient theocracies, the Pharaohs saw to it that medicines and drugs were regarded as sacred, and their knowledge was limited to the specially trained physician, many of whom were temple priests. The ancient Egyptians even had "Sanatoria" within the complex of various temples for convalescing patients.

Thus it was from that millenarian kingdom of the Nile, from Egypt, that much of the arcane medical tradition which flourished during the Middle Ages and unto the Renaissance in Europe, originated. Cornelius Agrippa and his Alchemical contemporaries were well acquainted with all the excellency of Egyptian, Persian, Ethiopic and Indian learning. The accumulation of ancient knowledge that was catalogued by Agrippa in his writings on Occult Philosophy, included the Egyptian medical lore that was zealously kept within the Temple Mystery Schools. In old papyri he saw references to that 'Wasting Disease', the 'Crablike pestilence that slowly gnaws at the entrails of men'. There it was described as an *inherent* disorder and intemperance within the body, thought to be brought about by an excess or lack of earthly elements.

The 'wasting' condition alluded to in the ancient sources typically points to cancerous processes, which they thought to be caused by a superabundance of humours (body fluids) which become agitated and separate from each other; in that unnatural, separated state, *each one turns against and torments the body.* The objectives of the Occultic treatment of this fatal illness was to restore the balance and harmony between the humours or body fluids, which would in turn cease their attack on the body.

While in the French Royal Court as personal physician to Louise of Savoy, mother of Francis I, Agrippa successfully treated a wide variety of venereal and infecto-contagious diseases that were rampant among the aristocracy of the day, with the exotic and secret methods of the Alchemist. A number of patients suffering from malignant and rapidly proliferative tumours were cured by means of natural biological substances made from certain animal fluids or humours, which are combined with selected botanical extracts.

Due to the secrecy with which Agrippa sought to conceal his arcane methods, accusations about the "demonic" and "unholy" means he was using to achieve seemingly miraculous cures of the 'Wasting Disease' (Cancerous tumours), were aligned against him. His previous bitter encounters with the Catholic Inquisitor of Cologne which resulted in his banishment from Germany, and his own criticism of his patron, the Queen mother, served as incriminatory antecedents to his many envious detractors, who were fearful of his growing power and influence within the court. He was eventually imprisoned by orders of Francis I, and a few years later died in confinement at Grenoble.

Agrippa's copious Alchemical records, notes, diagrams and Occultic writings survive to this day in rare private collections and in the secret archives of the Mystery Schools. And even up to fairly recent times, it was generally thought that the records of most of his exotic, secret treatments and Occultic Alchemical cures that he successfully used in his day, had perished with him, or were destroyed in the many book-burning campaigns that the Medieval Church periodically instigated.

But the wily old Alchemist had prudently ensured that the voluminous body of his Arcane writings would survive the crass intolerance of sundry obscurantist forces, to emerge once more in all their timeless power and majestic beauty, for the ultimate benefit of mankind.

Chapter 4

Clinical Experience in South America

Héctor Valdés was visibly perturbed and restless. He admitted to a state of increasing confusion with the lack of news about his son. Julio Velarde should have arrived on Wednesday's Aeroflot weekly flight from the Peruvian capital, and today Monday, five days since, we had no word from him, nothing at all to indicate whether or not he had arrived in Jamaica. All arrangements were in place, so that upon landing in Kingston he would call the telephone number I had given him... but, nothing at all from that point. We both assumed that he was not on the flight, for whatever reasons, because of course, he would have signalled his arrival long ago. He would therefore be on next week's flight; or, so we thought.

I had decided to verify the situation by calling the Velarde Valdés home in Santa Cruz once more, only to be told by Julio's mother that he was in fact in Jamaica *since last Wednesday,* and that the reason why he has not contacted us yet was because *he had to go to Negril first.* Furthermore, he was travelling on an Argentinian passport under the name Mauro Echenique Borges.

When I passed on all this information to Dr. Valdés he became even more frantic, fearing that Julio must have been robbed and killed somewhere in Jamaica, for, what else could explain the five day silence of the young man in a strange island where he knew no one, and spoke not their language. And Julio Velarde's sole mission in returning to Jamaica would have been to pay the fine imposed on his father by the courts.

I had gone to the hospital section that is within the General Penitentiary responding to an urgent call from Héctor Valdés. Upon arriving there, I was told that my friend was being treated for hypertension and that he appeared to be severely depressed. He was under the care of Dr. Carlton Fraser, M.D. who was the official physician for the penal institution. After assisting the interviewing process between the patient and clinician, and ensuring that he understood the medical instructions given regarding medications that were prescribed for him, we went aside and again tried to analyze the situation with his son Julio, and the unnerving silence from him.

Eventually I agreed to ask my contacts in the underworld, the feared urban ghettoes of inner city Kingston, to try to locate one Mauro Echenique Borges of Argentina, who is supposed to be somewhere in a guest-house in Negril, on Jamaica's touristic north coast. Because, of course, we could not go to the authorities with an official complaint of this nature. Things would have to be sorted out privately.

There was a disturbing facet to the whole scenario, which I mentioned to Dr. Valdés... Why would his son have to go to Negril, even before getting in touch with me? I had my suspicions which I kept to myself. Three days later a courier came to me with the dramatic news that Julio (or Mauro) was located just a few hours ago, in a cheap, third rate hotel in Kingston, where he had been since two days ago in the company of two prostitutes he brought with him from Negril. He was in a drunken stupor and had on him a large sum of money.

Shortly after, Julio and his two companions were checked out of the hotel by our friends and taken to a safe house nearby. A trusted attorney arranged to have the fine paid out of the money that Julio had on him; we later arranged also, a private nocturnal meeting of father and son within the prison compound. And Julio insisted on bringing along into the prison, the two prostitutes whom he claimed had protected him and kept him safe while he was under the effect of the ethylic alcoholic vapours. One of these young ladies was a Haitian, by name Denise, who was temporarily "working" clients on Jamaica's north coast. She had with her a pet snake which she carried around her waist under her garments, as a waistband.

And that snake would alert her whenever anyone with 'evil intentions' came close to her, by moving restlessly as it senses the malevolent aura of the approaching person. It was of a non-poisonous variety, and she would place it with a little food and water on the bedside table while she lies on her bed.

My suspicions were confirmed when we learnt that Julio did not bring any money with him to pay the fine, but rather, he had brought *more cocaine* instead, and in the same manner as his father did... built into the soles of the shoes. He had gone to the guest-house in Negril where the American again bought the shoes from him.

Young and naive, yet recklessly brave, Julio Velarde was the typical spoilt, immature Latin playboy; he was obviously in need of a few jarring experiences that would bring him to his senses. He was very fortunate that circumstances had played themselves out the way they did. We ensured that he was on the next weekly flight out, and later on confirmed that he was back home all right.

And mothers in many South American countries would wisely counsel their young sons with the adage, "My son, beware of the Chilean Woman, the Bolivian Justice and the Brazilian Black, they are all equally treacherous". Young Julio did not heed his mother's warning, for he easily succumbed to the bewitching Chilean beauty in his wife Deyanira. She was a daughter of the tough slums outside of the sprawling capital of Santiago de Chile, where a harsh upbringing are the daily realities of its rough infancy. She had migrated as a young teenager with her aunt to the Bolivian capital of La Paz, but merely a year after, opportunity came calling in the form of a young drug entrepreneur of the boom-town of Santa Cruz who introduced them to important personalities in the local society.

According to Dr. Valdés, Julio's mother had instantly detected a subtle wantonness in her future daughter-in-law, but her young son was determined to marry Deyanira, who was six years older. And all these concerns swirled in the mind of Héctor Valdés, adding themselves to the already heavy burden of dealing with his current situation.

I realized soon enough that I was also acting as advisor and in some ways as therapist for my friend, who was obviously emotionally devastated by the series of calamitous events plaguing him for the past few months. He was indeed suffering from severe depression and his decimated self-esteem and bruised dignity would plunge him into dark moods and suicidal broodings. I tried to provide the optimistic and positive outlook on circumstances, encouraging and inspiring him to just hold on a bit longer, for improvement and positive change might be near, and so on.

To achieve even a measure of success in those surroundings would be nothing short of miraculous. For Héctor Valdés had in fact descended into a phantasmagoric netherworld of incredible brutishness, a separate community which like an ancient fiefdom runs under it's own quaint code of rules. In the late evening hours, the main hall in the hospital ward would be manned by a skeleton staff of one or at most two guards who would be very congenial and friendly to these moneyed drug-offences inmates.

Inside, the heavy, pungent cloud of smoke was a truly cannabinated nicotinerama, and the whole area reeked of the pungent odour of marijuana and the sickly, chemical-laced residue of stale, burnt tobacco, which clings tenaciously to your clothes and burns the nostrils. And that hospital section within the General Penitentiary which was a fenced-off area of the large multi-acre penal institution, was populated not with the ill among the inmates, but with the privileged, with the occasional delinquent son of the local oligarchy, or the relative of a political warlord or perhaps the scion of one of the old plantocrats, for these all have a potent stranglehold on the 'commanding heights' of the island-nation's economic and socio-political life.

And all these Latin 'drugs-men' as they are called, had ample moneys with them and were frequently visited by their foreign and local friends, so, they are invariably located, whether they be ill or not, in that special section. But they had opportunity to tour the other areas of their enclosed citadel, and beheld as in a time-warp, the incredibly barbarous and filthy conditions in which the local prisoners are kept.

The medieval dungeon that passes for a penal facility was truly a museum piece, a stark reminder of the harshness and utter desolation that was the life of African slaves in Colonial Jamaica. The whole infrastructure was exceedingly decrepit and ancient, with its galleries of cubbyhole cells that were more like catacombs because of their incredibly small size. Built to contain exactly one adult who can stand or lie only in a north-south direction, these little cubicles were crammed with either three or sometimes five hapless wretches who would take turns at lying down to sleep, taking care not to overturn the small filth bucket they all must share.

What really startled and frightened the touring 'barons' was the fact that these mini-cells did not have a steel-bar door on them but instead a heavy wooden-plank of a door with old iron swivels and fasteners which would effectively entomb the captives within. An archaic system of a ratcheted, long iron brake would be drawn by a lever at one end of the line of cells, locking all doors there at one time. The heavy and surprisingly tough wooden doors ensured total darkness inside; there was a small cut-out at the bottom of the door for a metal platter of food to be pushed under, and also a small round peephole at eye-level for guards to look in periodically.

And these touring Latinos became acutely aware of their good fortune in not being placed right in the midst of the dark ages, complete with all the trappings of darkest plantation-days Jamaica. They saw and understood historically, why was it that the facility was located virtually in the heart of down-town with its northern gate towards Tower Street, and its southern gate right at the edge of the coastline on Kingston harbour. For up to recent times prisoners were transported to the infamous General Penitentiary by boat, and unloaded just there, at the massive rear entrance of what locals ominously term, the "workhouse".

As the days and weeks passed on, Héctor Valdés gradually began coming to terms with his present status. He started developing a clinical interest in his strange surroundings, analyzing the many aspects of aberrant human behaviour that daily made themselves manifest all around him. And there were numerous hopelessly pathological cases of mental illnesses, some of which began there, in that primitive milieu of appallingly subhuman conditions they are plunged into. Some of the half-crazed zombies seen walking around were victims of their own greed and addiction, many going through extended months-long psychotic episodes after smoking marijuana that had been deliberately mixed with the powdered tail of lizards, which has strong psychotropic and neurotoxic effects.

Others sustain serious brain injury resulting from the savage beatings that were regularly inflicted upon the inmates, by sadistic guards who clearly experienced quasi-orgasmic pleasure upon watching the pathetic flailings of their helpless victims who are often benumbed with intense, racking pain. Sporadically they would be brought, sometimes on a stretcher, some poor broken body with severe multiple traumatic injuries, perhaps for attempting to escape, or for some other relatively minor infraction of the rules.

On several occasions the congenial and knowledgeable Prison Medical Officer Dr. Carlton 'Pee Wee' Fraser would converse with Dr. Valdés on a wide ranging series of medical and scientific topics; these were most cordial exchanges which I willingly translated back and forth as the lively and erudite brainstorming sessions were truly intellectually stimulating for us.

And Héctor Valdés' encyclopedic breadth of information was nothing short of amazing. He told us of surgical techniques used by some Amazonian Indian tribes of the region of the *Gran Chaco* near the Brazilian-Paraguayan border, who suture wounds by carefully applying the claws of large, jungle red-ants to the clamped wound, then cutting off the ants' head along with its claw which holds the wound together and eventually falls off when the cut heals without a scar. And these same Indians deliver by themselves the babies underwater in the river from a crouching position, which has recently been accepted as being a more natural and less stressful childbirth delivery posture.

The ancient occultic method of curing asthma in infants is also well-known and practiced by the indigenous peoples throughout Latin America. The affected child is placed standing with his back against a young growing tree, and a lock of his hair is cut into the bark of the tree, but it must be done not with a sharpened knife but with an old rusty one. It works instantly in immediately and permanently stopping the asthmatic bronchospasms. They also used the bark of one of the willow trees in a decoction for pain and fevers, this being the natural source of acetyl salicyclic acid (aspirin) which is now synthetically made.

The powerful anthelmintic (against parasitic worms of the gut) that is found in the dried flower beads of the *Herba Santónica,* was used for worm infestations after they roasted and powdered the seeds of the plant; they then made a tea from this. Ipecacuana and Ephedra which today form part of standard Pharmacopeias, have been used for centuries by these Amerindians of the vast stretches of jungles in the Amazonian basin; most respiratory afflictions of a congestive nature respond favourably to the active factors in these plants.

Of the more exotic practices and beliefs that Héctor Valdés told us about, there was this which I found to be most intriguing, especially because I had come across several references to it in ancient works on Occultism and Metaphysics. It is said that a newborn infant who was born with the placental membrane covering his face as a veil, has the gift of prophecy and psychic vision, and that his life is marked for momentous deeds among men. Also, that the placental veil thus, has the peculiar virtue of protecting ships at sea from any calamity; so, captains and mariners will pay handsomely for such, because when kept on board, it will guarantee safe arrival of ship at port, no matter what the vessel encounters on its voyages.

And Héctor Valdés expounded to us in great depth and detail the true features and wide implications of the consumption of Cocaine by America and Europe. For, in the pre-Columbian era, during the early consolidation and expansion of the empire of the Incas, the Coca shrub had not yet been identified nor had its qualities been discovered.

With the perfidious treachery of the Spanish *conquistador* Francisco Pizarro whom with his swift abduction of the Inca king Atahualpa, and his later execution of the king even after obtaining for ransom a roomful of gold in payment for the life of the monarch, the vast expanse and wealth of the empire of the Incas had fallen squarely and securely into the hands of that small band of a few hundred intrepid adventurers taking possession of all that their covetous eyes could see.

The tremulous and superstitious Incas received the Spaniards with the reverence due to these 'white gods' whom their oracles had foretold would come from beyond the seas. The awesome superiority of firearms, the mounted cavalry upon the horse which was seen as a strange beast half-man and half-horse in one, plus the sheer bold resoluteness of the Europeans, easily cowed and subdued the natives.

But the rebellious and indomitable Inca prince of the aristocratic lineage of Atahualpa, on seeing the terrible demise of his father who was publicly drawn and quartered by four horses pulling on his limbs, fled the empire's capital of Cuzco, high in the Peruvian Andes mountains, to take temporary refuge in the sacred city of the Incas, the legendary Macchu Picchu, a solar-worship stone village hidden amidst the towering mountainous cliffs of a deep gorge, making it almost totally inaccessible to outsiders.

There, amidst the many temples and sacrificial altars where innumerable victims were immolated to the solar deity, Tupac Amaru communed with his ancestral divinities, seeking a revelation that would help him comprehend the terrible tragedy that had befallen his people with the arrival of the murderous white strangers in their big ships with the thunder of the fearsome cannons on them.

Merely a few days after, the prince was told that he must soon leave the refuge of Macchu Picchu's sanctuary because the invaders were moving in his direction. And he moved on, further and further on, until along with a few trusted companions he reached the western edges of the sacred Lake Titicaca on the high plains of what is today Bolivia. Exhausted and emotionally distraught, Tupac Amaru rested his tired body and quickly fell asleep against the trunk of a shrub nearby.

And he saw in a vision a celestial being of dazzling luminosity and beauty which said unto him... "The plant you are leaning against is sacred unto thy people, let them chew on the leaves for endurance and to eliminate hunger and thirst... *it shall be a blessing unto the Inca, but a curse to the white race."* He woke from his slumber and at once chewed on the leaves of the Coca shrub, and his servants also did eat of it, and they continued their trek eastwards to the jungle refuge where they would remain for many moons until the realm is delivered of the white demons who emerged from the ocean.

The vast empire of the Incas at the height of its development covered all that area stretching from southern Colombia unto Ecuador, Perú, Bolivia, part of western Brazil and northern Chile. And the tradition of the mastication of Coca leaves and the brewing of tea from the leaves for gastrointestinal disorders, is part of the folklore of the local indian population of these territories; and in the markets of Perú and Bolivia, it is quite legal to purchase the leaves from market vendors, but it is forbidden by law to process it in order to extract the alkaloid from its sap.

And the cocaine entrepreneurs, whether individually or in a syndicate or cartel, would themselves or through their agents, go deep into the Peruvian-Bolivian hinterland where the indian peasantry cultivate large stretches of the Coca shrub, and purchase cheaply huge quantities of the leaves which they pre-process right there in the jungle under cover of the deep and almost impenetrable tropical canopy of thick vegetation.

The local indians provide cheap and abundant labour, and they begin by digging out an enormous pit in the ground which would then be lined with plastic sheeting. Into the swimming-pool sized hole they would put a large amount of the Coca leaves, to which they add copious amounts of kerosene oil stacked there beforehand in stores usually holding a few hundred drums of that common petroleum distillate.

Over a period of several days and nights, those indian labourers methodically walk upon and stomp the mixtures of the leaves with the kerosene, in much the same way that Mediterranean peoples trod the winepress grapes with their feet.

The thin mineral oil, kerosene, gradually by its macerating action of mixing with the sap and fibres of the Coca leaves, transform the green mush into a dark brown glue-like paste, which after some evaporation is rolled into large basketball-size spheres of hardened gum. These large heavy balls are designated PBC (Pasta Básica de Cocaína/Cocaine base), and are loaded by the hundreds unto large cargo planes that daily lift off from their hidden jungle bases in Bolivia and Perú, on their trans-Amazonic low-level flight to well-protected landing sites in southern Colombia.

And about one-half of the Colombian national territory is under the effective control of the FARC (Revolutionary Armed Forces of Colombia) the leftist guerrilla organization which under the leadership of its legendary Commander Manuel Marulanda "Tiro Fijo" (Sure-shot), has been waging a relentless three-decades-long war of liberation against the Colombian government. Pacts of cooperation and protection with the liberation movements that still exist in many Latin American countries, have allowed the powerful syndicates of drug traffickers to move increasingly larger quantities of Cocaine into the North American market.

In precisely conducted operations, massive quantities of PBC bales are unloaded within Colombia's deep tropical rain forests near the border with Brazil, then transported deeper into the jungle interior towards the well-equipped laboratories where the refining process is carried out. Underground storage caves with large numbers of drums containing Sulfuric acid, Acetone and various catalyzers which are used in the chemical process, are well-stocked for continuous twenty-four hour manufacturing schedules. There, well paid, highly trained and qualified chemists and technicians proficiently subject the bales of Cocaine paste to the action of powerful organic compound solvents, acids and binders, to finally reduce the original mass into the alkaloid crystals commonly used as a narcotic.

A cortical stimulant, acting directly upon the cerebral cortex, it is highly addictive in susceptible individuals and moderately so in others. Addiction results when, with the availability of the drug, there is a personality problem such as the psychoneurotic disorder or a constitutional psychopathic inferiority. Psychoneurotic individuals ordinarily would use Cocaine to relieve their emotional or physical distress, while those individuals with personality disorders take it in order to enjoy their intoxicating effects.

The terrible sequela of ill-effects which invariably ensue with the chronic use of Cocaine hydrochloride are well known. From the emaciated bodies typically seen in long-term users due to poor nutrition, to gastrointestinal disorders, decreased libido or sexual appetite, to a breakdown of the nasal septum and cartilage and a variety of psychoses and acute paranoias in severe cases of Cocainism.

To Héctor Valdés, the current drug crisis that has developed in North America and Europe with the insatiable demand for the bitter white alkaloid which their young population voraciously consume, is an evident fulfillment of the ancient curse placed upon the conquering white race by the Inca deity centuries ago. For, curiously enough, cocaine addiction within the Andean nations of South America is minimal, contrasting starkly with the ferocious grip it has on the young soul of America's best and brightest.

60

But the American government's main concern regarding the national widespread addiction to Cocaine, is not really the effects it has on the population's health, but rather the massive transfer of *wealth,* the hemorrhage of countless billions of 'Coca dollars' which negatively tips their balance of trade, but more critically, places that vast amount of money with its attendant power to influence and corrupt, directly into the hands of outlaw drug-dealing organizations *over which they have no control.*

Dr. Valdés had lived for some three years in Colombia, in the border city of Cúcuta, parts of which fall within Venezuelan territory. There he learnt of the bizarre means employed by drug traffickers in the area. Because of the close links that exist between the peoples of both countries in the border region, there is much social and trade exchange as well as close family connections.

For many years, deceased family members to be buried across the border would be ceremoniously taken to Venezuela, complete in solemn funeral procession following the hearst. Routinely and with much deference, the cortege would be quickly waved-on by officials obviously unaware that the dead body had been eviscerated and the entire abdominal-thoracic cavity stuffed with up to forty-five kilograms of Cocaine. He had seen instances where cattle would have polyethylene bags of the narcotic surgically implanted in their abdomen or deep in the womb and birth canal, then to be driven across the border where the powdery implant would be removed.

And so, as varied and different methods of trafficking the illegal substance become known, other ingenious techniques are devised, and it matters not if it is eventually discovered, as long as it has some good probabilities of temporary or partial success, for, even at a meager 25% of safe market arrival, a handsome profit is made for all involved.

Héctor Valdés was convinced that drug penetration into the metropolitan countries could not be stopped and this was not because of the many alternating methods used by traffickers, but rather, because powerful transnational syndicates of drug organizations in South America had succeeded in developing virtually undetectable means of delivering huge volumes of Cocaine into the northern markets.

One of the larger cartels had for many years been funding secret research that a team of Chemical engineers were conducting, into the possibilities of achieving a 'molecular split' or bifurcation of the Cocaine molecule, its simple, non-structural formula being $C_{17}H_{21}NO_4$. A procedure was developed and demonstrated in prototype, by which the molecule was chemically separated into two component parts, each segment or part of the molecule no *longer having any of the characteristics of the original substance.*

This binary or two-part split of the Cocaine molecule, would allow the organization to easily admix each chemical portion into separate legal products, such as cosmetics, liquid or semisolid food preparations, and any of a whole plethora of common commodities which would then be exported openly and legally through the existing international trade network, separately. Upon arrival the two chemical 'halves' are again chemically treated, extracted from their temporary medium and recombined into their original structure and formula, thereby recovering up to 95% of the original volume processed.

The complex logistics involved in an enterprise of this nature would have proven to be daunting to the average large enterprise management team. But to the leaders of the shadowy underground syndicates and drug cartels, no idea is too far-fetched, no solution too outlandish and no vision too bizarre. The binary breakdown of the Cocaine molecule and its practical application to the huge commerce in illegal drugs, is quite likely in full operation at this time. The important consideration is not whether or not it will be uncovered, but rather, for how long will it successfully operate, before it ceases to be?

The pervasive culture of illegal drugs that runs deep and fast at all levels of the Bolivian society, and indeed, forms part of the popular folklore of the Andean republics of Colombia, Perú and Ecuador; gave the famous leaders of the drug cartels an aura of heroism and glamour, and many see them as crusading warriors inflicting demolishing blows to the oppressive colossus of the north who is helpless in the face of this peculiar form of psycho-social terrorism.

Dr. Valdés also told us of future, long-term plans of the drug cartels, that would enable them to face what is perhaps the greatest single threat to their continuing enterprise... the impending abolition of currency and all physical medium of exchange, to be substituted by an electronic identification number and computerized transactions at all levels. The overwhelming power and control that governments will have over every single citizen and their actions and choices, would make the large transnational commerce of the cartels impractical. Parallel systems are being considered by the drug lords as one of the many options to choose from. Other possibilities are rather more bizarre.

And as Héctor Valdés continued to adapt to his obligatory and depressing surroundings, it early dawned on him that any inmate who has money available in the prison, could easily obtain almost anything he wished for. Thus, many of them would arrange to have prostitutes or some other female friend brought into the compound at night for intimate activities. Others were taken out, escorted to spurious medical or dental sessions, then end up in bordellos or other distant locations along with their guard.

The vast majority of both guards and inmates consume regularly large amounts of marijuana, and to a lesser extent some 'hard' drugs too. And such a quantum of commerce in drugs take place within that penal facility, that, on occasions when the 'herb' is not available in the neighbourbood around, those outside users can easily purchase any amount from vendors within the prison, which is always well-supplied.

When next we met, Dr. Valdés shared with me some of his thoughts on the future plans he had been formulating for when he eventually regains his freedom. He was determined not to return to his native Bolivia, but to join his only sister in Colombia, who had been recently widowed. They had been very close from infancy, having grown up together into adulthood; Josefina Velarde who was four years older than Héctor, had married a medical researcher from Spain whom she met while studying in Madrid. They subsequently migrated to Colombia and settled there. Josefina Velarde de Cisneros had successfully completed her studies in Spain, eventually graduating from the prestigious Universidad de Salamanca with a Licenciate in Philosophy and History. She returned to her native Bolivia with her husband Dr. Axel Cisneros Vargas, but they shortly after went off to Colombia, where her husband was contracted to head a pharmaceutical manufacturing company.

They had settled in the small Colombian city of Pereira, south of Manizales in West Central Colombia, and were leading quite happy lives, with Josefina lecturing at the local university, while Dr. Cisneros became deeply involved in his work which allowed him to fully embrace the consuming passion of his professional life: research into the therapeutic effects of BRM's or Biological Response Modifiers on Neoplasms (tumours, metastatic or otherwise).

He had begun this work while he was in charge of the Research and Development department at a large biomedical enterprise in Spain which specialized in the preparation and manufacture of biological and hormonal extracts from natural sources. There was at that time a small team of three specialists working on the clinical, long-term assessment of a series of hormonal, placental and blood-fraction extracts and their effects on the growth, nutrition and reproductive processes of tumours, at the facilities under Dr. Cisneros' leadership.

The results of their decades-long investigations were little less than fully disappointing. There was not much previous work done in this area of biomedical research, although scientists had begun studying BRM's in cancer therapy in the 1960's, labeling the treatment modality, *immunotherapy*. After promising results obtained in animal studies, researchers initiated many large scale clinical trials to stimulate cancer patients' immune systems using the bacterial agents BCG *(Bacillus Calmette Guerin)* and C.

Parvum *(Corynebacterium Parvum),* but as the results of these trials were also discouraging, the research into immunotherapy as a possible modality for cancer treatment lost momentum.

The small team lead by Axel Cisneros had nevertheless persisted in evaluating a long list of biological extracts that were reputed at some time or other, to have anti-tumour action of some kind, but the results were consistently disheartening.

In his wife Josefina, Axel Cisneros had found a partner who in spite of her diametrically opposed specialty in the Classics and Philosophy, had developed a keen interest in her husband's work and in his idealistic quest for a natural, safe and effective anti-tumour agent which could prove to be the much sought after general systemic cure for most forms of cancer. She had taken the time to study into, and to try to understand the strange mechanics of tumour progression, proliferation, growth, vascularization for blood supply, enzyme mediated cell response, and many other aspects of tumour life and their causative factors. And as her interest grew and became as much a fixation in her mental life as it was for her husband, Josefina found that she was becoming more and more involved in the abstruse, arcane study of abnormal cells as manifested in the aberrant growth of tumours.

After remaining for three years in the Colombian-Venezuelan border region of Cúcuta, Héctor Valdés left for Pereira where he began working on the research projects that his brother-in-law was conducting. By this time, the investigations into the possible use of the BRM's in cancer therapy had gained momentum within the reduced circle of Dr. Cisneros' biomedical research team. The renewed vitality and focus evident in all aspects of the work, came about in an almost fortuitous manner, when in the course of independent historical research that Josefina Cisneros was engaged in, she came across detailed descriptions of ancient Alchemical procedures for the treatment of proliferative tumours.

She had been privileged to be given access to rare, unpublished manuscripts and correspondence dating from the fourteenth century, which were deposited in the private collections and libraries of several aristocratic old families in Spain. And Professor Josefina Velarde de Cisneros had undertaken to conduct an exhaustive research into the persecution and banishment of the Order of the Knight Templars which took place in the Europe of the Middle Ages; the work had been commissioned by the Grand Master of the local Masonic Lodge.

It was during the conclusive stages of the study, just about when she was preparing to draft the requisite report, that she encountered the surprising data. These were old Alchemical notations and descriptions of numerous procedures for the treatment of a long list of both, common and rare maladies of those days. Due to her familiarity with all manner of Philosophic, Occultic and Esoteric writings and lore, Josefina Cisneros was able to instantly identify the large package of musty old papers as the genuine renderings by scribes or copyists, of original Alchemical notations.

Dr. Axel Cisneros became very enthusiastic when he realized the potential implications of his wife's uncovering of that ancient information, and so, he at once started to consider the possibilities of a clinical verification of the Alchemical methodology for the treatment of tumours.

When Héctor Valdés arrived in Pereira, he found both, his sister and brother-in-law in a state of euphoria and heightened optimism due to the new direction that their lagging research efforts could now take. He was immediately made aware of the current status of their biomedical investigations, and the recent developments which promised to add an exciting new dimension to their so-far fruitless endeavours.

They convinced Dr. Valdés to join them in the project, as with his vast experience and knowledge there was much that he could contribute. Furthermore, they obviously preferred to work with someone who was connected by family links, because of the strict secrecy with which they must invariably surround their work. And numerous brain-storming sessions they convened; Héctor Valdés and the Cisneros' couple only, in which they formulated strategies, methodology and procedures to be implemented in the course of their planned series of clinical evaluations.

The material discovered by Dr. Cisneros' wife amounted to an extensive pharmacopeia of exotic botanical, mineral and animal biological preparations that were used by the Alchemists and Occult Physicians for the treatment of specific and well-defined morbid conditions. It also provided clear, direct and unambiguous instructions, detailing the proportions in which various substances, extracts and decoctions were to be admixed, their manner of administration and the duration of treatment. Strangely, there is no reference whatever to undesirable side-effects or contraindication to the use of these preparations in any of the documents uncovered.

They had all readily agreed that the voluminous manuscripts appeared to be genuine and that its contents describe in a categorical and forceful manner an entirely unorthodox approach to the treatment of both benign and malignant tumours. Dr. Valdés was quite impressed with the fact that all sources for the obtention of animal and botanical fluids, are readily known and quite commonplace in the tropical flora and fauna of the region. So, Hector Valdés and his sister enthusiastically encouraged her husband, Dr. Cisneros, to immediately begin working towards replicating, and therefore verifying, the astounding Alchemical data now in their possession.

Yet, in spite of the initial excitement they all exhibited in regards to their 'discovery', Axel Cisneros' brooding silence betrayed a kind of subtle doubt or discomfort within his mind... he appeared to be rather hesitant about the whole matter. His wife and brother-in-law did notice this seeming underlying concern, almost a trepidation in his sudden profound contemplation of what ought to have been regarded a heaven-sent bonanza.

And deep, within the hidden recesses of his mind, the searing memory of that harrowing psychodrama he experienced almost a decade ago, came back to haunt him with all the emotionally benumbing pain and helplessness he had sustained then. He knew well that he would never forget it, for, the devastating impact that unresolved guilts have on our minds inevitably colour and influence all our decisions and actions.

It was the pulmonary neoplasm (lung cancer) that was rapidly ravaging his maternal uncle, and had brought about intense sufferings and a renewed strengthening of old familial bonds, which had provided a uniting focus for the widespread old aristocratic clan of the Cisneros. The old man was afflicted with that form of cancer known as *Metastatic Carcinoma* which reaches the lungs secondarily from some primary location in the body. Due to the fact that the primary locus was not diagnosed and treated early enough, the condition had deteriorated to the extent where metastatic enlargement of cervical lymph glands and pleural invasion by the tumour was detected. It was subsequently established that the malignant neoplasm that had metastasized to the lung had emerged from a carcinoma of the stomach. The firm diagnosis was that of an extensive, inoperable secondary carcinoma of the lung.

Axel Cisneros had developed rather wide, international contacts with prominent members of the Oncological research community, and always endeavoured to remain in touch with them, primarily to stay abreast of the latest development in the field. This was a closely knit elite club where most researchers knew of the work that others were conducting, the particular areas of each other's interest and, generally the trend and direction that each group was pursuing. Of course, there were others too, highly skilled and trained individuals who were doing very sophisticated research projects for government agencies or for private industry, and whose work was conducted under cover of strict secrecy.

His uncle had been given a survival time of nine months, with the optimistic possibility of a maximum two years. He was undergoing vigorous radiotherapy to shrink the radiosensitive tumours, and was also being treated with the nitrogen mustard, mechlorethamine (HN_2), which produces transient general improvement and alleviation of distressing symptoms, with temporary control of pulmonary lesions.

The progressively increasing amounts of sedatives and narcotics that were required, undoubtedly pointed to a steady deterioration in his uncle's condition, and so, when a colleague in Italy offered to provide him with a steady supply of an experimental anticancerous bio-extract, he immediately accepted the offer. The substance which appeared to be a sort of colloidal suspension, had been tested in hamsters with remarkable results, and tests that were being conducted at that time on larger primates had not yet yielded results.

The patient was removed to a secluded facility where under Axel Cisneros' direct supervision, the mysterious therapy would be effected, meticulously adhering to the exacting instructions of the Italian researchers who insisted on their conditions of complete confidentiality for the trial. In this they were mindful not only of the pervasive illwill, envy and plain rivalry within the research community, but also of the medico-legal implications of conducting clinical trials on human beings with experimental and officially untested substances.

Arrangements had been made for the substance to be flown in by courier once a week, an exact and sufficient amount for each seven-day long therapy. The bio-extract was identified with the sole coded designation 'ZAM-1RO' and no other information was given as to its composition or source, or the proportional contents of its ingredients. It was however, obviously very unstable, with an extremely short half-life, since it would start losing its active potency within days of extraction from source.

Axel Cisneros shared with his wife and brother-in-law the emotional experience he had lived through with the experimental therapy that at his insistence had been used on the evidently terminal cancerous devastation of his uncle's lungs. He painfully described how the treatment regimen was carefully planned and conducted, and the almost immediate signs of improvement observed, which was in marked contrast to the merely palliative effects of the radiotherapy of the inoperable lung tumours, and the generally poor prognosis contemplated.

Just prior to initiating the 'Italian' treatment modality, clinical and laboratory findings had revealed that metastatic spread had been detected in the liver, the supraclavicular lymph nodes and the peritoneum. In spite of the dismal features evident in his uncle's condition, the attitude adopted by Dr. Cisneros and the immediate family was that "there was nothing to lose in trying something else".

Within six weeks the whole clinical picture started showing signs of definite improvement, with the invasive, destructive nature of the tumour appearing to retrogress. But, most important were the laboratory results, initially from the examination of pleural fluid for tumour cells and subsequently by the antigen-specific tests which revealed a progressive remission of cancerous cells. At three months of continuous administration of the ZAM-1RO the first 'negative' result from the oncological laboratory was received amidst the stunned elation of family members and medical workers.

Tests were repeated in order to obviate the possibility of false-negative readings, and almost constant monitoring of clinical features and vital signs along with the evident improvement in the general physical and mental condition of the patient, rubricated the pervasive relief and optimism felt by all concerned. And while Axel Cisneros was already pondering the numerous implications and consequences of the successful experimental procedure, and the worldwide effect that it was bound to have in so many profound ways, others were still trying to come to grips with the seeming miraculous cure they were witnessing firsthand.

One of the conditions imposed by the supplier was the requirement of a regular, twice-weekly clinical and oncological (laboratory) report on the progress of the clinical trial. The biomedical research facility in southern Italy had ensured that at all times they had the final word on critical decisions relating to the tests, and in fact had reserved for themselves an overall dominance throughout. They had in effect circumvented the strict regulations governing the testing of new biological and pharmaceutical preparations in their own country, by having the initial clinical studies done beyond their borders.

Of course they would still proceed with the lengthy bureaucratic formalities involved in having the bio-substance approved for testing in humans, but in the meantime the privately conducted test would yield *valuable preliminary data* which would help to determine whether or not they would proceed with the development, certification and subsequent marketing of the therapeutic product. At any rate, if the results of the private clinical trial are unsatisfactory, the project can easily be aborted; if on the other hand, results warrant pursuing product development, then, a significant advantage in terms of testing and development time would have been gained.

Axel Cisneros' uncle was in his early sixties, and had enjoyed a relatively healthy life. He was a burly, heavy set man of sober habits whose only known hobbies or distractions were his beloved chess game and the traditional 'corrida' or the bullfight, on which he served as one of the judges on most of these seasonal events. He was not in the habit of consulting regularly with the family physician, and would make efforts at concealing any minor symptoms or distress he might experience.

Some cancers in the alimentary tract are hopelessly advanced before they cause sufficient symptoms to bring the patient to the physician; furthermore, symptoms of gastric cancer, which was the primary and discrete locus of Dr. Cisneros' uncle carcinoma, are entirely non-specific and include either singly or in combination, a variety of symptoms such as: vomiting, anemia, occult blood in the stool, anorexia, upper abdominal distress, usually but not necessarily worse after eating, all of which may be indicative of other conditions. It was only when the many vague and non-specific complaints, typical of many patients with gastrointestinal cancer, were becoming really troublesome and could no longer be hidden from family members, that the old man acceded to submit to medical expertise.

At approximately four months of continuous treatment with the experimental ZAM-1RO, the patient was exhibiting a most remarkable recovery; he was steadily gaining strength and vitality, eating and exercising moderately, and generally evidencing a thorough comeback which was supported by the continuing favourable laboratory results.

A visit by two clinicians from the Italian biomedical research institution, suppliers of the therapeutic extract used, served to confirm the success of the clinical trial. They returned home with various samples of blood plasma and other body fluids for testing, and again emphasized the agreed-upon proviso between the Italian researchers and Dr. Cisneros, that any public announcement regarding the clinical study and its results could only be made by the research institute at such time as they would deem appropriate.

A few days after the visitors had returned to their country, Axel Cisneros was informed that in light of the evident success of the treatment, the administration of the ZAM-1RO bio-extract would be gradually diminished until fully terminated. Frequent laboratory monitoring for signs of recurrent pathologies and keen clinical observation of the patient's condition was to continue, and reported to the research team in Italy.

The experimental treatment came to an end some four weeks after, but supportive therapies and a special dietary regimen was maintained... Then came the absolute shocker. The stunning report from the oncological laboratory was hand-delivered with a request for Dr. Cisneros to call them immediately upon receiving the results.

This latest laboratory report had the surprising disclosure of a peripheral blood picture suggestive of acute leukemia; they were also urging that diagnosis be urgently established by bone marrow aspiration. When Dr. Cisneros called the laboratory, they told him that they were already running parallel tests in order to verify the reported results, but they could not await these... urgent measures needed to be taken at once.

Deluded into a false sense of security by the previous series of encouraging laboratory results which had declared his uncle free of neoplasmic (cancer) cells, both he and the medical support team working with him, misdiagnosed as an acute rheumatic fever the apparently infectious process of sudden onset with high fever, and secondary infection of mouth, throat and lungs which had emerged. The faulty rheumatic fever diagnosis was further strengthened by the patient complaining of joint pains.

As his uncle's condition rapidly deteriorated, Axel Cisneros brought in an eminent Oncologist of considerable experience and clinical judgement, who at once noticed the tell-tale signs of moderate enlargement of liver, spleen and lymph nodes, along with the progressive weakness and pallor of the skin. He immediately began a justifiably bold therapy, placing the patient on a continuous Intra-Venous (I.V.) infusion of hydrocortisone... trying to elicit a satisfactory hematologic response. Though he knew that the remissions produced by these adrenal steroids are usually brief, lasting 3 to 6 weeks despite continuous treatment; at least it could buy the clinician, and the patient, some time during which other therapies may be used. He soon concurred with the preliminary diagnosis of an *acute leukemia.*

This rapidly fatal form of leukemia begins as a local proliferation of neoplastic cells arising in the bone marrow, the lymph nodes, or in other areas as the spleen and the liver. These cells are disseminated through the blood stream and infiltrate many of the body tissues. Because the immunologic mechanisms are impaired, there is an increased susceptibility to infections, and, generally the prognosis is one of an invariably progressive course which is ultimately fatal.

Axel Cisneros' colleagues in Italy had strongly advised against reinstituting the ZAM-1RO experimental substance in his uncle's condition. In spite of his many pleadings in lengthy telephone conversations, they firmly refused to be swayed on this, claiming only that they had to conduct further tests on the bio-extract they had supplied, in order to determine exactly why a relapse had occurred after the treatment had been suspended. They appeared to have no available explanation for that baffling turn of events.

His uncle's condition suffered a marked deterioration as the disease had become refractory or resistant to treatment, and in spite of strong supportive treatment with the use of blood transfusions for anemia and bleeding, and antibiotics to control infections, the patient soon succumbed to persistent anemia, hemorrhage and the intercurrent infections for which he had no natural defences.

And although Dr. Cisneros was emotionally devastated by the death of his uncle, he nevertheless tried to analyze and find answers to the many questions arising out of the series of unpredictable and nerve-racking events in his uncle's fatal illness. He agonized and revisited every step of the therapeutic course administered, but soon realized that there was no real alternative available, for they had ventured into the 'terra incognita' of experimental pharmacodynamics where often the clinician is forced to make swift decisions entirely based upon his sole judgement... without reference to any previous experiences... a lonely exercise in subtle intuitive hunches.

The laboratory tests were conclusive, and the initial tendency to hope for a remote error or procedural shortcoming in the many tests conducted, were soon enough set aside when they confirmed the results by separate, independent biomedical laboratory. Yet, the nagging mystery of the initially deceptive lab results along with the supportive clinical evidence objectively observed and assessed at bedside seemed to mock their efforts at elucidation. Then came the subsequent sudden relapse, and the reemergence of the generalized neoplastic disorder with its monster cells infiltrating most of the tissues of the body with a fulminating viciousness bordering on a kind of genetically ordained vengeance of the mutated cells upon its human host.

Amidst the inevitable soul-searching, recriminations and self-doubt that he underwent, many theories, rationalizations and mere speculative explanations, suggested themselves to his confused and bewildered mind. He thought it likely that with the presence of the experimental bio-extract ZAM-1RO effecting its still unknown mode of anti-cancerous action, some of the neoplasmic cells or a "cell-actuating" or "activating factor" responsible for their emergence, might have migrated to some remote or inaccessible area of the body, there to remain asymptomatic and dormant, perhaps under cover of a temporary mutational form not recognized by the experimental substance.

And so, the only firm conclusion he could safely arrive at, was that his uncle's terminal illness did respond initially to the experimental therapy, and that the laboratory tests had confirmed at one stage the total abscense of neoplastic cells in his body, in fact declaring him free of cancer. And there was also the dramatic clinical improvement of the patient right up to the time when the treatment was ended. Yet still, it failed. And the cruel certainty of that fact with its many unresolved questions and dilemmas, continued to haunt him through these many years.

That harrowing experience had certainly shaken Axel Cisneros' self-confidence. It had done so, to the extent that he developed a pathological fear of failure, and was now given to lengthy procrastination, profferring excuses and stalling decision-making processes and the taking of strong action in urgent situations. A pervasive fear seemed to colour his every decision, and all his actions were too carefully weighed before venturing forth on a chosen path.

Both his wife and brother-in-law had listened attentively to the surprising disclosure that Dr. Cisneros had made, sharing with them for the first time, what to him was truly a mind-bending and gut-wrenching experience of intimate pathos which he kept hidden in the folds of a subjectivity long accustomed to a defensive infolding of personal pain and persistent sense of guilt.

The catharsis of sharing that long-suppressed spiritual burden did have a salutary effect upon him, for he felt strangely relieved, sensing a kind of widening of the encircled limit he had placed around the memory of that stark event, as he candidly brought them into the subjective world of his fears, doubts and yearnings.

And as they understood and sympathised with him, trying to encourage and strengthen the pioneering and adventurous disposition that as a researcher he was imbued with, he confided that the underlying fear he had regarding the ancient Alchemical anti-tumour bio-extract they were planning to replicate, was: Could it be that the ZAM-1RO substance which was used with fatal results in his uncle's case, was the same as the Alchemical extract they were now about to develop and clinically test? If so, wouldn't they be about to trod upon that same path of success and eventual failure he had lived through, nine years ago in Spain?

Certainly, it was virtually impossible for them to ascertain the origin or composition of the Italian experimental substance due to the extreme secrecy with which the suppliers routinely surrounded their work. Furthermore, they all knew that a request for samples of the ZAM-1RO extract would be denied, since this could only be for analytical purposes, very much in breach of their security regulations. The only option available was to develop and clinically test for themselves the reputed Alchemical antitumour biological preparation, a course of action which would have to be conducted clandestinely in conditions of total confidentiality since it would involve therapeutic clinical trials on human beings, albeit terminal cancer patients.

Early on in their deliberations, the Cisneros couple and Dr. Valdés had decided not to seek the assistance or collaboration of anyone within the cancer research fraternity, as they already had signalled in numerous ways their total antagonism and outright hostility towards any independent investigator working in the field. The old, long established rivalries that pervades the scientific community would be further exacerbated by the fact that the Cisneros-Valdés team was pursuing their investigations within the unorthodox and little-understood area of Alchemy and Occult Medicine, a realm for which the establishment had a visceral antipathy.

But, by far, the most critical decision they had to make was in respect of the clinical trials that would have to be carried out. The ancient Alchemical documentation in their possession outlined therapies 'in vivo', that is, the treatment of cancerous tumours directly in human beings without reference to previous testing in animals. After much deliberations they concurred with Héctor Valdés' proposal to conduct the trials directly on humans afflicted with hormone-mediated and virus-mediated terminal cancer.

During those lengthy brainstorming sessions, their going the 'Maverick' path by directly experimenting on humans, was rationalized by contrasting it to the infamous Nazi-German grotesque and barbarous series of 'medical' experiments carried out on countless Jewish, Gypsies and Slavic death camp inmates.

At the end of the Great War in 1945, the voluminous medical records and the thousands of morbid pathology tissue samples that had been obtained from concentration camp inmates who were deliberately infected with a wide variety of infecto-contagious diseases, were taken over by allied occupation forces, and subsequently delivered to selected research centers in the USA, England, France and the Soviet Union. There they would serve as most valuable 'medical-scientific' indicators of human physiologic tolerance parameters, which current ethical and legal prohibitions on human experimentation, would render difficult if not impossible to obtain.

The results of many thousands of these horrendous Nazi-era 'experiments' have been, and are still being used, by NASA (National Aeronautics and Space Administration) in the USA, as "Human borderline tolerance indicators" in designing the equipment, technical apparatus and space suits used by their astronauts, as well as for the planning and structuring of various experiments during manned space flights.

Thousands of macabre and diabolic 'medical-scientific' procedures were carried out on the helpless victims of German physicians and research scientists. Ghastly sterilization operations, castrations, fiendish tortures, deliberate starvation, percutaneous absorption of toxic chemicals, were among many authorized procedures recorded in detail in theatre registers of surgical operations at well-known German universities of Hamburg, Heidelberg, Wurzburg, and scores of other medical and research centers. Some camp medical records document up to 4,000 of these 'experiments' at just one such location.

The 'medical' works of German physician Dr. Joseph Mengele, a.k.a. 'The Angel of Death' on heredity, morphology and physiology of identical twins and the chilling mutilations and tortures he visited upon death camp inmates at Treblinka, Auschwitch and Bergen-Belsen are well known. There, extremes of temperature, heat, cold, traumatic pain, mechanical pressure on body tissues, stretch resistance of body limbs and tissues, resistance to noise, thirst, hunger, extremes of drowning times in both sexes and upon adults and infants, sterilization of women by x-rays and by pumping toxic chemicals into the uterus, were round-the-clock routine procedures.

In order to determine the lowest (and the highest) temperatures that humans can tolerate, concentration camp inmates were immersed in cauldrons of progressively hot or cold water, and their physiological reactions to various temperature levels as well as the relevant time factors before death, were methodically recorded. Extremes of pain tolerance, dehydration, starvation, sleep deprivation and electrical shock were later on expanded to include exotic experimentation on snake, spider and scorpion venom effect on humans, and these are just a few of the unbelievable catalog of nightmarish atrocities that in the name of 'medical science' these Frankenstein doctors of Nazi Germany practiced upon countless thousands of their death camp inmates.

And, although the dreaded Nazi SS 'select troops' were the ones charged with the mission of carrying out the Hitlerian 'Final Solution', it was the concentration camp physicians who had total sway and final authority in the selection of individuals as subjects for their bizarre and sadistic 'medical' experiments. Yet, the physiological and pathological data that resulted from all these criminal procedures, have been and are still being used by many renowned research centers in government and private industry, as well as in Academia where much of the German 'scientific' findings appear in respected medical texts still in use.

Dr. Axel Cisneros had finally agreed with his wife and with his brother-in-law. They would replicate the Alchemical anti-tumour procedure, scrupulously following the detailed instructions as they appear in the ancient writings, although the quaint and obsolete terms used in the old, medieval Alchemical manuscripts, along with the mysterious arcane symbology typical of the Occultic Arts, made the interpretation of the minute procedural instructions given, extremely difficult and laborious.

According to an analysis of origin carried out by Prof. Josefina de Cisneros, the Alchemical manuscripts were from the period called *"Iatochemistry"* which was the era when chemistry was applied to the study of medicine; she had correctly given an estimated date of around the 13th century, with portions of it directly attributable to such eminent Alchemists as Roger Bacon, Albertus Magnus and Raymond Lully. Their works had been exhaustively compiled by Cornelius Agrippa a century and a half later.

The planning stage of the project which they had already named "ZAM-2RO", was completed in little over one year. All technical aspects of the clinical trial had been incorporated into a carefully outlined 'Manual for Clinical Study – ZAM-2RO' in which a stage-by-stage procedural guide would direct every step of the project right up to its culmination.

Héctor Valdés assumed the responsibility of directly super-vising the meticulous process of extracting the series of designated plant sap which would be subjected to a number of processes such as filtration, stabilization and sterilization of the fluids, as well as the subsequent combination of these in specific proportions. The end product is then stored in opaque containers in order to prevent light affecting the potency and stability of the admixture which is highly photosensitive.

It was after weeks of tedious and painstaking efforts that a moderate amount of the botanical extracts was accumulated and carefully maintained at an optimal temperature to preserve its integrity. The traditional methodology called for an admixture 'in vivo' of the combined plant-vegetable extract with the secret animal humoral fluid.

This latter biological ingredient demanded very specialized and close attention, both, in its extraction procedure as well as re-garding its subsequent handling and administration. They had learnt that this, the principal component for the powerful Alchemi-cal anticancerous compound, the animal secretion concentrate, should not be stored due to its marked instability and extremely short half-life, as it begins losing its effectiveness within 24 hours after being separated from its host.

Due to this peculiar characteristic of the most critical fraction of the ZAM-2RO fluid combine, the collection of the secretion must be done at a location which is relatively close to the clinical trials site. Furthermore, the whole procedure of extracting the animal-source bio-substance had to be structured in such a way as to ensure that a continuous operation yielding a steady volume of the bio-substance, without interruption, is achieved. Dr. Cisneros, perhaps reminiscing on the sad experience he underwent with his uncle's terminal illness, had emphasized the absolute necessity of securing a reliable supply of the humoral extract, because, in the course of the projected series of clinical tests they envisioned, it was indeed imperative that an inexhaustible source of it be constantly available, in order to maintain 24-hour uninterrupted therapeutic blood levels of the compound ZAM-2RO in every patient participating in the clinical trials.

The Cisneros-Valdés team was acutely aware of the marked antagonism and bigotry that the international Cancer research establishment has consistently displayed against any probability of the discovery (or re-discovery) of a natural-source cure for cancer, for this would definitely endanger the massive multi-billion dollar industry of early detection with its various invasive modes of treatment now being used. And so, they easily concurred with the obligatory necessity of protecting their investigative work by a strict cover of secrecy. Later on, anticipating potential success, they would decide how to, and when to, reveal the results of their work to the world.

Because the old Alchemical parchments did not outline a specific method for collecting the animal humours or fluids, Dr. Héctor Valdés had to design a special extracting catheter which would draw moderate fluid volumes from the creature *without killing it.* With this peculiar specification the ancient Occultists surely wanted to prevent the contamination of blood, tissues and body fluids and humours with the adrenaline-like secretions occurring in many animals undergoing sudden acute stress or near-death episodes.

While these preparations were taking place, Professor Josefina de Cisneros continued her in-depth examination and analysis of the old parchments with their extensive and amazing scope of information on all manner of Occultic and Alchemical treatment and quaint procedures. In them, reference was made to several prominent Alchemists of the 8th and 9th centuries who resided in the courts of the Caliph of Baghdad, and whom, under the influence of Chinese Alchemists had postulated the concept of the 'Philosopher's Stone' then regarded as a 'medicine' that could turn a 'sick' or base metal into gold and also act as an 'elixir of life' or universal cure for all diseases.

Among these ancient sages the most notable were Jabir ibn Hayan (721 – 815 AD) author of a number of Alchemical treatises, as well as the Persian Occult physicians al-Razi (886 – 925 AD) and Avicenna (980 – 1036 AD). They, along with other Arabian Alchemists had discovered new chemicals such as the alkalis and the process of distillation. Their works had had a marked influence on the famous Occult Physician Paracelsus (1493 – 1531), who was the first in Europe to mention zinc and to use the term 'alcohol' to refer to the spirit of wine. It was the Arabian Alchemists who discovered that by heating the compound iron sulphate, they could produce "Oil of Vitriol" which is known today as sulphuric acid, and they could also make compounds such as potash and sodium carbonate. They had also identified the elements Arsenic, Antimony and Bismuth.

Josefina de Cisneros never ceased to be surprised at the vast quantum and profound complexity of the knowledge that had been acquired by these medieval practitioners of the Sciences. The Alchemical explanation of the nature of matter was particularly thought-provoking and curious. To the Alchemist, matter was thought to have a 'soul' which could be transferred from one element to another by means of the Philosopher's Stone, and this Alchemical concept was included in the treatises of such scholars as Arnold of Villanova, Albertus Magnus and Roger Bacon.

Paracelsus had, however, postulated that the principal object of Alchemy was the cure of the sick by ensuring a bodily 'balance' of the three elements: salt, sulphur and mercury, which when present in the body in the proper proportions would give health. These concepts prevailed for many centuries until they were superseded by the modern ideas and discoveries into the nature of energy and matter. The period of Alchemy, though, lasted for a very long time, that is, from the beginning of the Christian era to the 17th and 18th century, and during that time, most of these notions enjoyed currency and acceptance in the spheres of Sciences and learning.

And while his wife delved deeply into the Arcana of the ancient Occult physician, Dr. Axel Cisneros was holding a series of preliminary interviews with the relatives of a young lady in her early twenties who at that time was undergoing intensive treatment for inoperable brain cancer in the United States. She had previously been treated in Germany and in France by the most prominent Oncologists there, but her condition had deteriorated to such an extent that a decision had been made to transfer her to the U.S.A. where the usual invasive forms of therapy were immediately instituted.

Maritza Romero Hernández was the third daughter of a widowed major cattle rancher in northern Colombia. Her mother had died four years before of complications following radical hysterectomy (total removal of the uterus) for endometrial cancer. Maritza herself, had for the past eighteen months been suffering from the terrible side-effects that the massive radiation and chemotherapy treatments had brought about in her already weakened body. She was severely emaciated and had lost virtually all her body hair, including eyebrows, lashes and even nostril hairs.

The American cancer centre had wisely informed the family of the extremely poor prognosis in her case, as the estimated maximum survival time for Maritza had been set at between four to eight months, and there was very little that they could do for her at that stage, apart from merely providing palliatives for temporary symptomatic relief, until the inevitable fatal outcome takes place.

She had earlier exhibited the classic triad of tell-tale symptoms, (headache, nausea and vomiting, and choked disks) usually due to increased intracranial pressure. Later on, periodic convulsive seizures accompanied by psychotic episodes, drowsiness, lethargy and a general impairment of mental faculties confirmed a preliminary diagnosis of a deep occipito-parietal brain tumour. Tumour cells had subsequently metastasized, spreading to adjacent areas and obstructing ventricular pathways.

The family physician that had originally attended to Maritza was aware of the research work on cancer therapies that Dr. Cisneros had been conducting for the past decade and a half. When he mentioned this to the Romero Hernández family, they immediately decided to contact Axel Cisneros to see whether there was any possibility of helping their ailing daughter. And although they fully understood the experimental nature of these natural Biological Response Modifiers, and were aware that it had not been tested in humans within recent times, they readily agreed to have Maritza undergo this treatment modality, in a desperate bid to save her life.

******

Héctor Valdés gradually came to the realization that the experiences he was going through in Jamaica were undoubtedly of some value, for, in spite of the markedly unpleasant and repulsive character of the odious environment in which he found himself immersed, there were at times, the occasional light moments, and even those incredible, truly unbelievable episodes of mirth and human folly, which unexpectedly bring with them a welcome respite from the stultifying routine of daily depravity and human misery typical of prison life.

It was indeed a sort of compulsory learning experience for him, a veritable 'tour de force' into the more squalid manifestations of the human pathos, which, if he managed to survive it, would definitely enrich his understanding of the sorry human condition. He was finally adopting a philosophical view of life's circumstances, that vital combination of mental or temperamental traits and resources which equip a person to deal with such extremes of adversity and dehumanizing indignities as those he frequently saw at Jamaica's General Penitentiary.

A bit of distracting excitement occurred with the latest rumour making the rounds in the prison grapevine. Early morning talk among the inmates at the prison's hospital section related the overnight escape or 'disappearance' of a prisoner from one of the security blocks, an event which was not discovered until the early-morning daily muster, or counting of heads. A general search of all areas in the institution failed to locate the 'escapee', while the police dragnet carried out in surrounding neighbourhoods yielded no positive results. Even one week later there was no sign or news whatsoever of the missing inmate.

The totally wall-enclosed facility had within it, a separate walled-off inner area which was used as a female prison and which was staffed by a cadre of female prison guards. This sub-section remained effectively disconnected from the larger male-populated areas, segregating and totally keeping apart the two sexes.

Stunned disbelief in some, outbursts of laughter and even applause by others joined the speechless embarrassment of prison authorities, when it was discovered that the escapee did not really flee the prison, but was for all of ten days carefully hidden, fed and amorously nurtured by the female prisoners in their walled-off section, to which he had arrived by crawling through connecting sewer mains.

The ensuing hush-hush investigation revealed that the 'escaped' male convict would have continued enjoying the lubricity and pneumatic bliss of countless sexual encounters with most if not all of the rotund, sex-starved lady prisoners for many more days, or weeks, had it not been for the 'toothless old hag' who blew the whistle on him after he refused to also 'service' her. This whole incredible happening led to the abandoning of the women's section there, and the subsequent relocation of the female prison to the old English colonial gaol of Fort Augusta, on the shores of Kingston harbour.

84

Commenting on this incident, Héctor Valdés explained that in Bolivia, and in many other Latin American countries, regulations stipulate that when a prisoner escapes confinement, the guard responsible at the time is immediately taken into custody to serve the remaining sentence of the escaped inmate, until he is recaptured, at which time the guard is then released. Because of this rule, upon the escape of a prisoner, the responsible guard also flees and goes into hiding until the escaped one is found, at which time he resurfaces to reclaim his position.

Shortly after, there was the curious incident of a prisoner from the Cayman Islands who was serving time at another Jamaican penal institution, the dreaded Saint Catherine District Prison, located some 18 miles from the capital city of Kingston in the old township of Spanish Town. It was in the early hours of the morning, shortly after midnight, that the guards at the General Penitentiary's main gate were awakened from their slumber by a loud and insistent knocking on the outside of the massive wooden gates. The Caymanian prisoner whom they knew well from his previous sojourns there, was vociferously *demanding to be let in;* he had just escaped from the St. Catherine District Prison because he could not stomach the food there nor the 'bad treatment' he was getting. Not knowing anyone in Jamaica, he opted for the only place where at least he had some 'friends'.

He was of course readily admitted, and a telephone check revealed that authorities at the other prison were not even aware of his departure. He was allowed to remain at the Kingston facility where he later held court with the other inmates in true 'press conference' style, narrating how he did not have to walk the full distance, but flagged down a passing police patrol car, since he was in his own civilian garb, telling them how he was robed by thieves and wanting only a ride into Kingston. He was dropped off in the vicinity of the General Penitentiary, and was even given some small amount of money by the sympathetic patrolmen, promising them to make a formal complaint at the police station during the day.

And so, the periodic occurrence of these and many other instances in a seeming unending series of unbelievable tragic comedies of official buffoonery, often provided the welcome relief from the daily drudgery of his present miserable existence. Of course, that meeting with his son, albeit within the prison, did much to his morale and lifted his spirit to new heights of resilient endurance, a condition of mental fortitude sorely needed by Dr. Héctor Valdés in his present situation.

In all this, there was an eerie kind of emotional detachment that I noticed in his general disposition, particularly when he spoke about that period in his life during which he was involved in the biochemical and clinical research work carried out by his brother-in-law in Colombia. I got the distinct impression that with the death of Dr. Axel Cisneros, just as he was preparing to present the results of his research and clinical findings before the Swedish Academy of Sciences, both Héctor Valdés and his widowed sister Josefina de Cisneros, had become discouraged and to some extent, had even lost some interest in the work.

It was as if he could only concentrate on the immediate urgencies of daily survival, and in the unending and repetitive planning and constant reviewing of the numerous scenarios he visualized for his still nebulous future. And, although he had in his possession a significant portion of the biochemical and clinical records, histological and cytological studies results, laboratory reports and hundreds of photographic slides and prints showing 'before' and 'after' shots of patients who were successfully treated with the experimental ZAM-2RO alchemical compound, he seemed not to be placing much hopes in either continuing the work, or in presenting their joint experimental clinical studies to the international scientific and medical fraternity.

Both, Héctor and his sister Josefina, were convinced that only Dr. Axel Cisneros could have made a successful presentation of their work in Stockholm. Only the Swedes, and a Japanese university, had responded with any degree of interest to the first tentative contacts made, and after some reciprocal communications, an agreement had been arrived at with the Swedish organizers for a comprehensive clinical study report to be made before a designated committee of the Academy. They felt that the deceased researcher was the sole individual with the required professional qualifications, skill and research experience, along with the unique clinical experimental trajectory that would enable him to command the respect and acceptance of his scientific peers.

A few weeks later when I next saw Héctor, he was enthusiastically engrossed in translating some technical pharmacology and therapeutic papers in Spanish and Portuguese, that our friend Dr. Fraser has received from México and from Brazil. After a while our conversation gravitated towards that same topic of the Medieval Alchemists' discoveries, and their secretive means of treating various malignancies and proliferative tumours. This was a subject which my friend was always willing to discuss openly.

On this occasion, Héctor summarized the many theories and speculative concepts that the Cisneros-Valdés research team had evaluated in the course of their pioneering work. Virtually all of these ideas and tentative hypotheses, some of which are accepted today as valid in explaining the cause and origin of the emergence of neoplasms in their many manifestations of Cancer, have their 'counterpart' in the medieval principles postulated by Alchemists and Occult physicians.

There was, for example, the arcane concept of a "trans-generational" propensity in certain individuals to cellular mutational changes, which the ancients ascribed to a reincarnatory stigma or a pronounced Karmic imbalance. This in turn, demands a restoration of that vital balance between the negative polarity of 'nous' (the earthly or material elements in our bodily composition) and the positive polarity of 'nous' otherwise known as the VLF, Vital Life Force. This latter positive polarity is an ethereal, energizing force of indeterminate nature present in the air and which combines with the negative or 'spirit' earthly elements, through the medium of the adhesive magnetic attraction that keeps our cells and body parts together.

The ancient sages knew that the Vital Life Force or positive polarity of 'nous' enters the body of a newborn through the mouth and nostrils at time of birth, when the first breath is taken. With the sudden expansive action of air in the lungs saturating the alveola, the VLF is disseminated through every cell, accomplishing the total, independent vitalization of the newborn, now beginning its autonomous phase of life separated from its nurturing host, and no longer dependent on the reduced level of VLF supplied by placental blood.

They also conceived the 'adhesive magnetic' force that adheres our cells to each other, as critically important in the maintenance of health, and any weakness or alteration in the subtle qualities of that physiologic magnetic force, inevitably brings about any of a wide variety of pathological states, one of which is the emergence of the feared malignant proliferative tumours. Therefore, hunting and the slaughter of animals, or humans, creates an adverse Karma in the individual which affects the physiologic balance of his body *at the cellular level.*

The practitioner of Occult Medicine had an awareness of the effects of the subconscious mind upon cell life. They believed that if subconscious promptings or urgings are ignored or suppressed, then, vital imbalance is intensified and organisms and cells alike react by mutating to cancerous forms. They were very much aware that certain mental attitudes and emotional states such as depression, anxiety, panic states and sustained or prolongued fear, affects hormonal production and balance, which in turn have a marked influence on leucocytes (white blood cells) and the immune mechanisms of the body, thereby frequently rendering the subject open to the profound cellular transformations characteristic of cancerous processes.

They had also recognized that it was these selfsame profound cellular transformations, usually triggered by abnormal genetic alterations, and which made malignant cells more sensitive to radiation, at the same time cause them to proliferate and reproduce seemingly unrestrained.

Both, radiation therapy and chemotherapy – in the latter of which there are over 100 drugs available, usually used in combination of two and up to ten different drugs at the same time –

are forms of symptomatic cancer treatments that are intensely aggressive and invasive, generally destroying innocent cells along with the targeted neoplasmic ones.

It was these inherent therapeutic shortcomings of the standard cancer therapies that had stimulated the search for alternative modes of treatment within the realm of the natural biotherapies. And so, after much preparations and with limited resources and support, they embarked on the quiet, secretive clinical study in which three cases initially of manifestly terminal cancer would be treated with the alchemical preparation ZAM-2RO.

Agustín Romero Hernández responded swiftly and positively to the requests and conditionalities stipulated by Dr. Cisneros, placing a large tract of unused ranchland along with suitable structures and installations, at the disposal of the research team. The remoteness and isolation of the site proved to be ideal for the purpose, and so, within a short time, equipment, provisions and a small cadre of technical support workers were all placed to start the experimental clinical study.

In his account of that truly exciting period of his recent past, Héctor Valdés painted a mesmerizing picture of the tense and demanding atmosphere that prevailed at "El Sanatorio"; that's the name that his sister had optimistically given the heavily wooded jungle-green enclave they would call 'home' for the next six months at least.

'Don Agustín', as Maritza's doting father was called throughout the vast cattle and coffee domain of the region, commanded enormous influence and power with all and sundry. His inherited wealth came from the centuries-old Bolivarian aristocratic family, the Romero's and the Hernández's who were in control of extensive tracts of fertile farmlands and thousand-heads herds of cattle. To this they had added, through shrewd investments and corporate business deals, an even greater economic strength and sheer liquid resources.

It was said that the Romero Hernández family kept most of their wealth safely tucked away in European banks due to the socio-political instability that has plagued Colombia through many generations. One of his sons had been kidnapped by dissident leftist rebels, and later released in exchange for a huge ransom, an episode which caused him to greatly increase the moderate security measures previously set for himself and his family. This pronounced security awareness was most evident at "El Sanatorio", where heavily armed 'farmhands' and 'assistants' ensured an almost total isolation and quietude for all those involved in the quasi clandestine endeavour of testing an ancient and obscure preparation of uncertain origin and composition on human beings.

Don Agustín had eagerly and efficiently facilitated whatever was necessary to carry out the treatment, and concurred with Axel Cisneros' suggestion that the clinical trials be conducted with at least two other patients, terminal cancer cases as well, in order to broaden the scope of the test, but also to satisfy the need for parallel observation and clinical contrast and comparison. What Dr. Cisneros did not mention to Maritza's father, was the fact that his daughter's clinical picture was so dismal that a very poor prognosis with inevitable fatal outcome had been discreetly agreed upon by the clinicians. Thus, the perceived need for other, more 'promising' cases so as not to consume valuable bioextracts on her seemingly hopeless terminal pathology.

Both Dr. Fraser and myself saw, through the vivid descriptions painted by Héctor Valdés, the simple yet very functional outlay of the rather spartan facilities at El Sanatorio. The main and larger building was set against the dugout side of a rounded hill; its eastern half was entirely given to the 'clinic' where a properly appointed hospital section contained four beds with a separate support and equipment area. The western end of the structure, divided from the medical section by a large common area, was the living quarters for the research team of three with two technicians.

The outstanding feature was, however, the extraction and processing unit which was located at about 800 meters from the clinic and living areas, and were connected to each other by a narrow pathway through the heavy shrub and vegetation. There was only a medium size warehouse-like building there, and some 100 meters behind it could be seen some enormous wire cages with a few dried trunks of trees therein, upon which were perched many vulture-type birds, while others fed on cattle carcasses and assorted carrion. The putrid scent emanating from that repulsive aviary could be noted from many kilometers around.

Maritza had been accompanied by her father on the trip to the exotic facility. They travelled in a private ambulance driven by one of Don Agustin's trusted men, and on the way she was being constantly encouraged and comforted by her loving father who sometime after would confess that on that journey he struggled with a brooding feeling of finality and tragedy for his beloved daughter.

The other two patients were already at the facility. They were a 63 year old gentleman with advanced prostate cancer who had been undergoing radiation, chemotherapy and hormonal treatments, after the standard surgical methods had failed to arrest the spreading of the disease. He had been given only 14 months by his doctors and was quite willing to try anything that would offer the slightest hope, whether a cure or perhaps merely a prolongued survival time beyond the one year dictum of his physicians.

The other patient was a matronly mother of four in her mid-fifties who had been battling a bilateral lung cancer for the past three years, and who after receiving up to 28 radiation treatments and five rounds of chemotherapy was still afflicted by progressively widespread cancerous metastases of the lymphatic system and recently emerging neck tumours. Her case pointedly confirms the often seen situation where traditional chemotherapy quickly loses its effect on cancer cells while unleashing its destructive power on healthy cells.

These two had already been receiving a single dose of the bio-extract compound every twenty-four hours; this was supported by a strict dietary regimen, constant monitoring of therapeutic blood levels and clinical physiologic signs. Regular Antigen-specific and cytologic laboratory tests were routinely done by an external biomedical laboratory in the city, to which twice-weekly blood and fluid samples or biopsies tissues were sent.

Shortly after arriving, Maritza was also placed under the ancient anti-tumour regimen which would run an expected course of two phases lasting ninety days each. As Dr. Valdés explained, a selective saturation and cellular binding of hyperimmune factors in the ZAM-2RO compound would effect a kind of 'strangulation' or cellular 'starvation' of all neoplasmic cells wherever in the body they may be found, bringing about *the seeming magical alchemy of a complete obliteration of cancerous malignancies* with consequent restoration of health in the patient.

Although the mechanism by which the alchemical compound would achieve its selective destruction of cancerous cells was not fully understood, the researchers knew that there was some form of 'transfer of immune capabilities' involved; what was not yet determined was the duration of anti-tumour activity once the compound was withdrawn, and more critically, whether or not there was any kind of permanent or semi-permanent transfer of a heightened immune activity which would allow the patient's own bodily defences to effectively ward off future proliferation of mutated 'monster' cells. For the time being, resolving these questions were beyond their immediate objectives; the research trio knew that a clinical cure backed by confirming laboratory tests would be most welcome by everyone involved.

And although they did not anticipate any legal problems emanating from the experimental treatment, care had been taken to obtain carefully worded signed documentation from the families, releasing the researchers from any liabilities regarding the clinical trials to be carried out on their desperately ill relatives.

The Cisneros research team estimated that the alchemical bio-extract would have to be tested in at least twenty advanced cancerous cases, before any definite conclusions could be arrived at in respect of the efficacy and safety of the arcane biotherapy. They surely would not encounter any major difficulties in securing suitable subjects, as the rapid increase in the incidence of terminally ill cancer patients ensured that a grim pool of 'hopeless' cases was always available. Their principal concerns were rather more prosaic, since the reaction of an intolerant and envious scientific establishment had been consistently negative not only in respect of discoveries and new developments by their own colleagues, but especially so when an 'outsider' gains recognition for some pioneering work within any of the mundane sciences.

The other consideration they had to carefully weigh and bear in mind was the unorthodox and abstruse, occult character of the whole methodology employed in the biotherapy, as well as the surprising source of the biological extracts used. The latter they had decided to conceal not only from the patients and their families, but even, as much as possible, from the technical and support workers at the clinical site.

It was after twenty days of meticulous administration of the ZAM-2RO alchemical compound, that unexpected signs of slight improvement in the general clinical picture of the first two patients was observed. At that time Maritza's condition could only be classified as 'stable', as there was yet no indications of tumour remission. The team was however, heartened by the fact that there were no signs of reactive intolerance or untoward side effects in any of the subjects, while analysis of body fluids and transudates revealed an almost total absorption of the biocompound.

That almost imperceptible, almost subclinical hint of improvement in the two older subjects, gave the team a most welcome stimulus and their first real indication that there could be some substantive basis to the medieval claims of the Occult physicians, and that their alchemical methods could be replicated and applied successfully in the battle against the much feared malignancies of mutated monster cells.

In respect of Maritza Hernandez's guarded prognosis, they could take comfort in the fact that the clinically evident intumescence, (the swollen, enlarged intracranial tumour) was showing signs of a subtle reduction, although there was a persistence of the intracranial pressure and cerebral edema.

During her course of radiation and chemotherapy treatment in the United States, the consulting neurosurgeons in attendance had even considered the possible usefulness of a radical pioneering procedure, a Hemispherectomy. This operation involves the removal of a brain hemisphere, (half of the encephalic mass), and is carried out usually to cure intractable seizures; later on, through the process of "plasticity" the remaining mass of the brain takes over the functions of the missing hemisphere. In Maritza's case, the aim would be to arrest the aggressive and rapidly proliferative malignant lesion, but that potential course had to be abandoned due to the evident widespread metastases of the cancerous cells throughout most of her body. At this, the eleventh hour in her ebbing life, it was felt that the total systemic anti-tumour action of the alchemical ZAM-2RO compound, would eventually obliterate every single malignant cell. The lingering question was... Was it too late? In two weeks time they would be able to say.

When, at the daily evening meetings they held, Dr. Cisneros announced that there were now a total of nine other potential candidates for the clinical trials, both Dr. Valdés and his sister Josefina were elated and voiced their excitement at the prospect of expanding the range of the tests, He, however, cautioned them against any premature exuberance because it was still too soon for any firm anticipation of success, and, furthermore, there was a number of daunting obstacles still ahead of them.

And, surely, that small, anonymous research team at El Sanatorio, working a strange amalgam of modern medical science mingled with the alchemical art of the ancients, realized fully that their bold biomedical adventure constituted more than a mere mocking of legal pedantry, and that nagging element of very serious risks for both patients and clinicians was constantly on their minds.

For, not only were the patients chancing an abrupt reduction of their medically estimated survival time by substituting the unknown alchemical method for the standard anticancer treatments, but they were also risking an even more immediate death through a possible adverse reaction to the compound, probably caused by the mechanism of organ or tissue rejection. Then also, the potential consequences to the researchers-clinicians in the event of failure were too daunting for them to even contemplate.

Legally, there was the almost unthinking adherence by the courts of justice to the many insidious, archaic modes of obsolete jurisprudence with its numerous ricocheting analogies, which would surely level accusations of criminally reckless conduct that endangered the patients lives, plus the whole ethical-moral considerations regarding the experimental nature of the treatment which the team administered to humans without any kind of official or medical sanction. They did not, however, dwell too much upon the many other consequences of a personal, professional and even social sort which would inevitably follow in the wake of failure... Yet, amidst these and other intimate, subjective mental storms each of them battled in quiet desperation, they nevertheless found renewed strength to continue in their rare quest for one of nature's most jealously guarded secret. And the clinical trials at the remote and rustic El Sanatorio, continued, and the team persisted in maintaining the strict therapeutic regimen bequeathed unto them by the ancient masters of Occult Medicine and the Alchemical Arts.

****

The intensification of the illegal drug commerce between the production centers in South America and the lucrative markets in Europe and North America, continued to spin off a steady stream of imprisoned traffickers into Jamaica's archaic penal structures. As most of them were Latin Americans who tended to cling together in captivity, Héctor Valdés managed to keep abreast of the latest happenings in the international drug culture sub-world.

From the Colombian captain who had been caught along with his five crew members, he had learnt that the notorious head of the Medellín cartel, Pablo Escobar, had ordered an all-out war of nerves and terror against the government in an effort to dissuade them from extraditing any Colombian citizen to the United States on drug charges. The relentless campaign of urban bombings, assassinations and kidnappings was rapidly discombobulating the already fragile fabric of that divided nation, slowly stifling under the oppressive strangulation of a centuries-old moribund oligarchy.

And as the bombs wreaked their indiscriminate shower of fleshtearing nails, nuts, bolts and lead into the bodies of unsuspecting innocent shoppers and passersby in Colombian cities, and the feared "Sicarios" (hit-men) pumped hails of bullets from their swift motor-cycles into official vehicles halting at traffic lights, it was the selective kidnapping for ransom or 'prisoner exchange' of wealthy individuals, which had the most profound effect on the society.

The Romero Hernández clan were no strangers to the vagaries of life, security and survival within their dangerous milieu. They had had their baptism of sorrows with the abduction of Maritza's brother a few years ago; that at least ended after he was released some six weeks later with the payment of a sizable ransom to his captors.

It was merely seven months after, that a similar but much more tragic episode impacted upon the unfortunate aristocratic family. Maritza's flamboyant maternal uncle had long been on the target list of one of the many splinter leftist guerrilla groups plaguing the rich coffee cultivating area. They had been closely monitoring his every movement for close to a year, but were unable to get a clean hold of him, for, he himself and every other member of his family were under the protection of burly private security agents.

All this heightened state of alertness among the wealthy clan came about after state intelligence agents attached to Colombia's dreaded secret police, the DAS (Departamento Administrativo de Seguridad/State Security Bureau), warned the family that leftist guerrilla elements were planning to kidnap at least one family member. The rebel's opportunity came unexpectedly one day, when Maritza's aunt-in-law, her uncle's Mexican-born wife, Electra Abrego, was on her way to the airport accompanied by two bodyguards, one of whom also drove.

Their vehicle was intercepted by heavily armed men who dragged her out of the car and proceeded to riddle it and the two men inside with a shower of bullets. The attackers then pulled out the lifeless bodies of the two men, and with a razor-sharp machete inflicted upon each cadaver the well-known trademark wounds of Colombia's drug underworld: the "merino" cut, by which the head is severed from the body with one swift semicircular swipe, and the 'necktie" cut, when the tongue is pulled through a deep gash in the throat and allowed to hang as a tie.

This was meant to be a clear message to the wealthy landowning clan. The guerrillas were deadly serious and would stop at no evil or extreme of depravity to achieve their objectives.

It was not until three weeks later that the insurgents demands along with dated photographic proof that their victim was still alive, was received. A sizable ransom had been paid, but even after seven months not another word had come from either captors or victim; then, unexpectedly, news reached them that Electra had been found. She had been set adrift in a dugout canoe on the river Cauca which flows north from the Andes mountains into the Magdalena river; at this confluence she was brought ashore... she was still heavily drugged... they had also sent her back in an advanced state of pregnancy.

And so, everyone in the region knew that it was this devastating experience that had impelled the Romero Hernández clan to become closely connected with the shadowy right-wing paramilitary organization, the feared MAS (Muerte a Secuestradores/ Death to Kidnappers). Manned by off-duty secret police and selected soldiers, this ruthless and unforgiving death squad wreaked their chilling brand of rough justice on the urban cadres of left-wing insurgency groups who had developed into a fine art, the craft of the kidnapper. Well-financed by leaders in business and industry, they went about methodically hunting down any and every known operative or even sympathizer of the rebels, visiting ghastly mutilations and dismemberment on their victim's bodies.

And as the vicious circle of Colombia's blow-for-blow retributory vendettas among her many armed groups continued unabated, the deeply superstitious and fatalistic people in this bastion of Roman Catholic 'culture', looked on with dismay and perplexity at the series of uncontrollable events that were threatening to plunge the nation into another chaotic whirlwind of violence and bloodshed.

All this background information on Maritza Romero Hernández's family history had been obtained through many hours of interviews between Dr. Cisneros and members of the clan. He was exploring the possible links between the emergence of Maritza's cancerous tumour and the time when major traumatic events with a strong emotional content for her, had taken place. He had received recent biomedical research results on psychological toxins which accumulate in the body as a consequence of sustained major grief or trauma and which can trigger the cancerous transformation of cells. It was also believed that these psychological toxins had a marked damaging effect upon the immune system. Since the immune system must ward off and neutralize the cancer cells which are being formed in our bodies on a daily basis, any reduction in the protective activity of this vital immune mechanism can lead to the emergence of malignancies.

Meanwhile, the production of cocaine in Colombia had reached astronomical levels, and in the last four years had doubled its tonnage and expanded its market penetration in metropolitan countries. And, although United States anti-drug aid to Colombia had reached unprecedented levels, up to $1.5 billion a year which is among the highest US foreign aid in the world, and up to 200 American special forces are currently helping to train Colombian forces in anti-insurgency warfare, the war is being lost to the rebels and the US risks becoming involved in a widespread civil war in Colombia.

Official sources both in Colombia and in the United States recognize that there are still at least 15,000 persons in Colombia alone, involved in producing and exporting Cocaine to some 430 drug organizations in North America and Europe. And this worldwide international network has proven to be, not only highly sophisticated in its operational methodology, but also ruthlessly brutal in its unstoppable objective of achieving global status for its evil commerce.

And the deleterious effects that the quasi-industrial productive structure of the noxious and highly addictive narcotic substance has had on the socio-economic an political life of Colombia, is undeniable. From the corruptive penetration of billions of "narco-dollars" at the very highest levels of officialdom, the judiciary and big business, to the popularity of the "Bazuco", a residue of cocaine processing that is cheaply available to poor urban youths, who smoke it for its psychotropic pleasurable effects, no segment of Colombian society remains untouched by the coca-industry.

Paradoxically though, the secretive biomedical cancer researchers in the remote hinterland, felt themselves vastly removed from all the violence, misery and intrigues that were commonplace in the haemorraging South American republic. They continued, stoically labouring at their delicate and abstruse craft, holding fast to the hope that nature would finally yield the curative secret that the ancient alchemists claimed to have pried from her tightly clenched fists. Then...

At the El Sanatorio facility, two more patients were added to the number of subjects undergoing the experimental treatment. Beds and additional equipment were brought in, and a renewed sense of guarded optimism seemed to energize the team members, for now at last they were seeing definite signs of clinical improvement in each of the patients, including Maritza. They were however, awaiting results of the battery of antigen-specific tests from the laboratory; they felt confident that the results would reflect a heightened level of immune activity and the beginning of remission of the cancerous process.

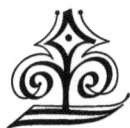

Illustrations

The Alchemical and Hermetic Rose Cross

This intricate symbolic representation is a very old mystical symbol. The cryptogram is composed of two Rosy Crosses united into one. The small Rosy Cross at the center point, representative of man, (the microcosm), is in turn the center point of a larger rose residing at the heart of the large cross, symbolic of the universe (the macrocosm). Upon the four ends of the large cross are inscribed the three Alchemical symbols; Mercury, Sulphur and Salt. At the top of the cross, Mercury is placed in the center, Sulphur on the left, and Salt on the right. Upon the other ends of the cross the symbols appear in such an order as to conform to the esoteric tradition.

Also upon each arm, adjacent to the Alchemical symbols, is the symbol of the pentagram, wrongly called five-pointed star, representing the victory of the quintessence over the four Alchemical elements.

The wheel at the top of each pentagram represents the quintessence; the small triangle on the left with the point downwards and a line parallel to the base symbolizes the earth; the triangle above with a line parallel to the base but with the point upward, represents the air. The upper triangle on the right of the pentagram with the point downward symbolizes water, and the lower small triangle on the right with the pont upward represents fire. On the lower arm of the figure, below the large rose, is an hexagram (the so-called six pointed star or Star of David) and is composed of two interlaced triangles. At its points are inscribed the six planets according to the ancient astrological tradition: at the bottom is the moon; at its right is Venus, followed in turn by Jupiter, Saturn, Mars and Mercury. At the center of the hexagram is the Sun. The order of arrangement of these symbols conforms to certain Kabbalistic rituals.

The lower end of the longest arm is divided into four sections by two diagonal lines according to Malkuth of the Kabbalistic "Tree of Life". The four sets of three rays, which extend outward from the center of the large cross, symbolize the Divine Light. The letters upon each large center - ray combine into INRI, representing the Latin maxim meaning, "Nature is completely renewed by fire". The letters upon the smaller rays represent invocative names of Latin, Egyptian and Greek origin. The petals of the large rose on the cross are twenty-two in number, and stand for the twenty-two letters of the Hebrew Kabbalistic alphabet. At the center of the large rose is the microcosmic Rose Cross, an unfolded cube with a five - petalled rose at the center. Four barbs emerge from this smaller cross, pointing into the four directions in space.

This complex "encyclopedic" symbol was the "Key" of the Alchemical arts, encoding with its majestic power and beauty, the cosmic laws that govern man and his world. Also encrypted within its arcane symbology is the secret LOGOS or creative word by which both, the visible and invisible world came into being, according to the traditions of Hebrew Kabbalistic numerology.

EL LOGOS

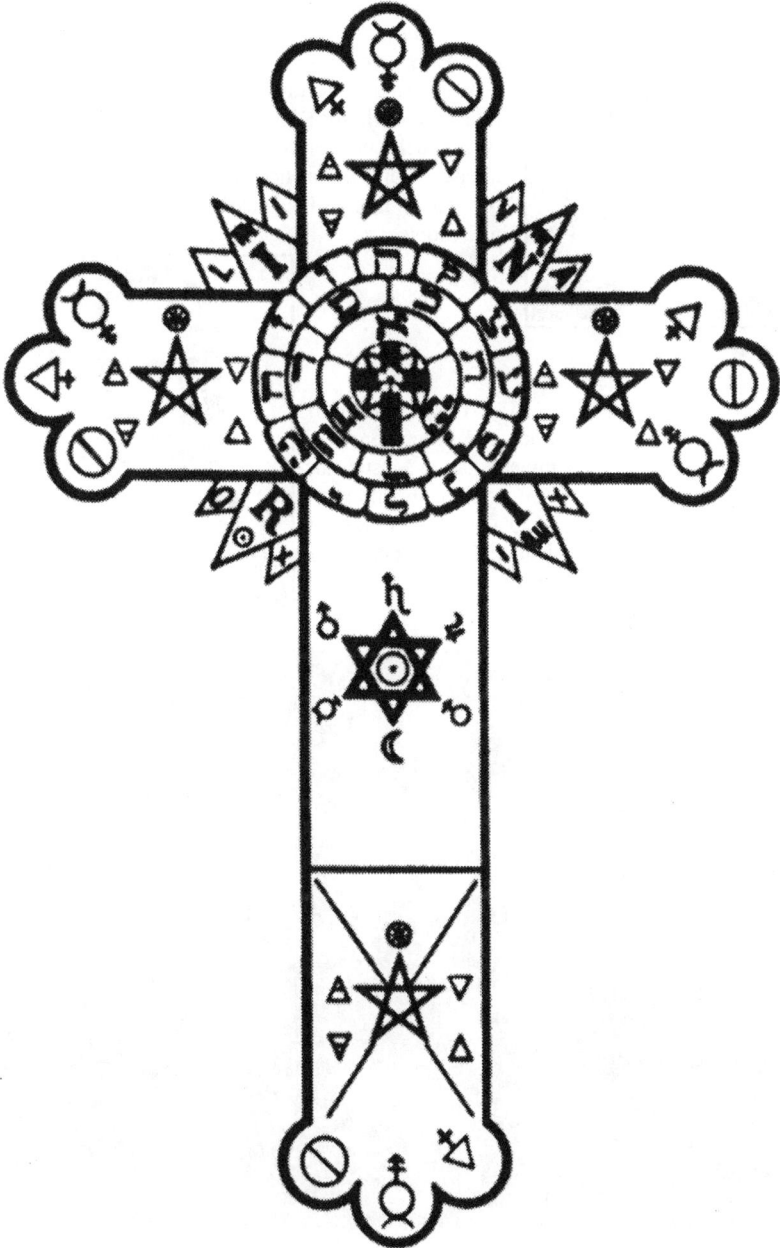

The Alchemical and Hermetic Rose Cross
(by kind permission, Supreme Grand Lodge, AMORC)

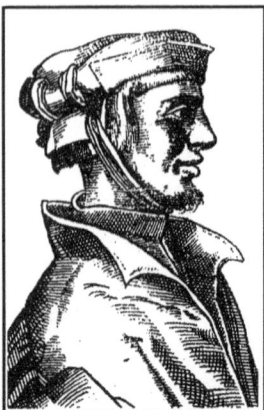

[1]Cornelio Agrippa von Nettesheim (1486-1535); from a 1527 engraving by an anonymous artist. Philosopher, Alchemist, Physician, Theologian, Military entrepreneur and acknowledged expert on Occultism. By alchemical means he transmuted fourteen tons of lead into gold for King Charles V of Spain and routinely cured cancer, epilepsy and febrile diseases. Branded as an heretic and imprisoned by orders of Francis I, he died in confinement in Grenoble.

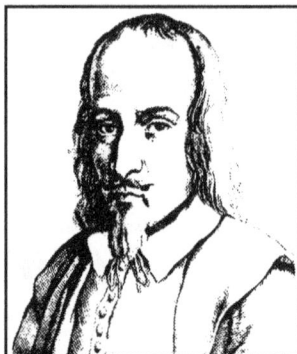

[2]Jakob Boehme (1525-1624). German mystical philosopher and practitioner of speculative Alchemy and nature Mysticism. Known as the "Philosopher shoemaker" Boehme's writings had a profound influence on later intellectual movements. (Courtesy of Staatsbibliothek Berlin).

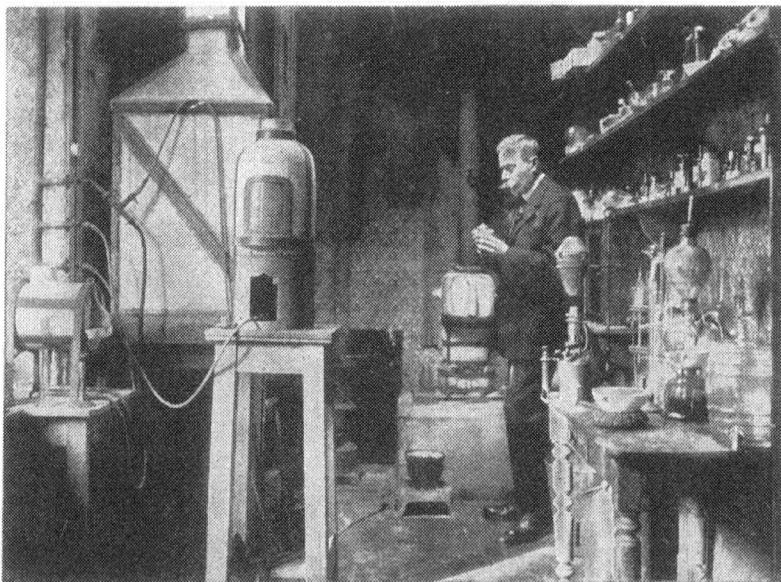

[3]A modern Alchemist in his laboratory. M. F. Jollivet Castelot, Past President, French Alchemical Society and High Officer of La Rose Croix of France. He demonstrated the Alchemical principles and produced gold by transmutation of base metals. (Photo, courtesy of Supreme Grand Lodge of AMORC).

104

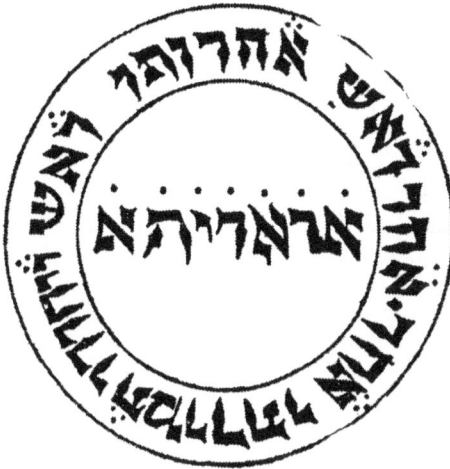

⁴Mystical talismanic figure by Sereno of Samos, used to cure the undulant fever or Brucellosis; it is worn around neck by the patient. (From Annals of Occult Medicine).

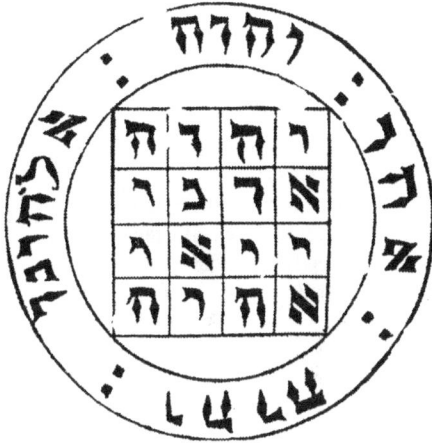

⁵*Araritha* Talisman against all illnesses, according to Rabbi Hama in the "Book of Contemplation". The foursquare names of God in Hebrew are inscribed upon virgin parchment with consecrated ink made from ash of Frankincense and Myrrh and Gum Arabic; it is carried on the person.

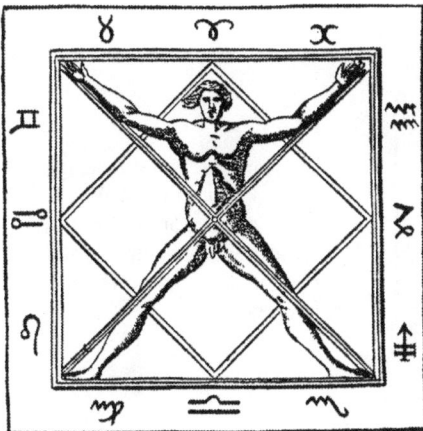

⁶Mystical proportions and harmony of the human anatomy; forming a *perfect square* with center point at the navel. (Annals of Occult Medicine).

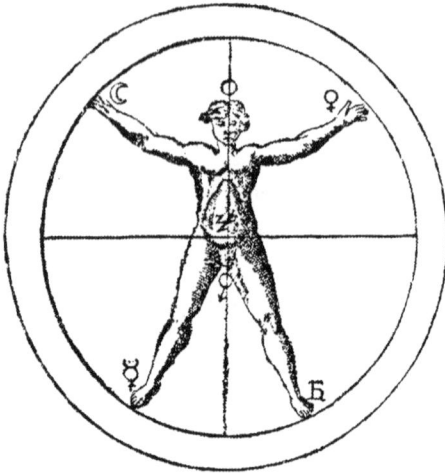

[7]Circle with center at navel and equilateral triangle formed by feet and penis.

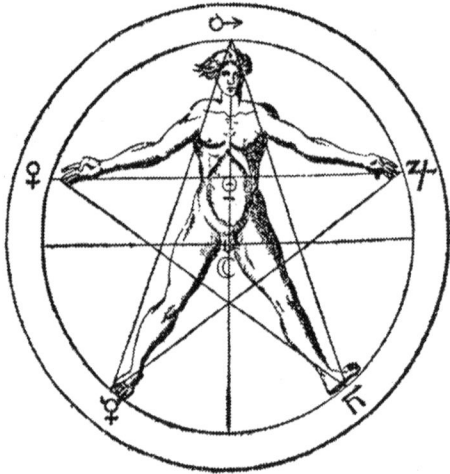

[8]Circle over top of head, and lowered arms with finger tips and feet on circumpherence. Such figure with center beneath the penis is divided in five equal parts making a perfect pentagram (five pointed star).

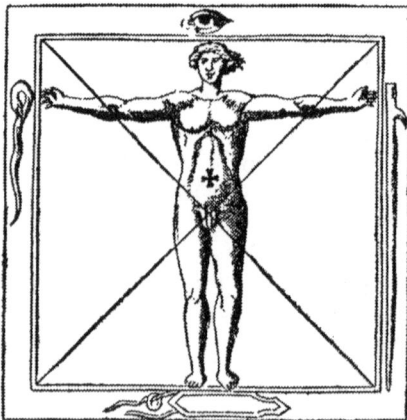

[9]The square measure also depicts a well-proportioned body. With feet beside each other and outstretched arms at the sides, man forms a perfect square with its center at the base of the penis.

106

Luna

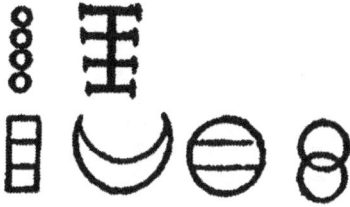

Mercurio

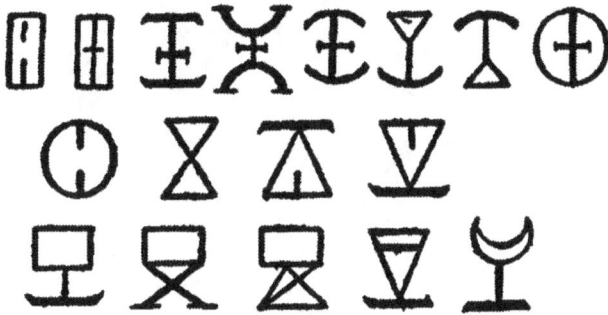

Venus

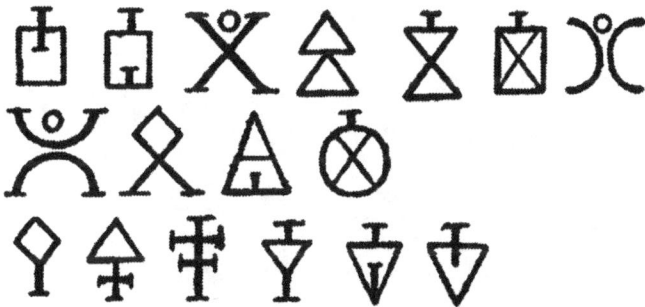

Sol

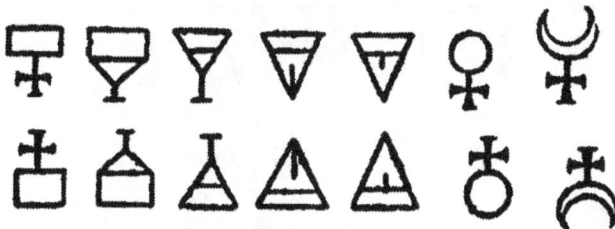

[10 & 10a]Alchemical Planetary symbols used by the Alchemist to formulate procedures and various experiments.

107

10a

Marte

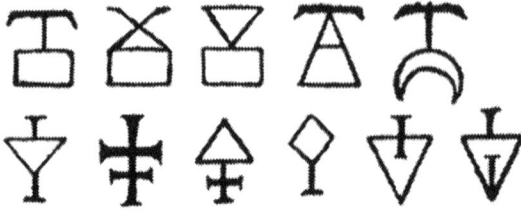

Júpiter

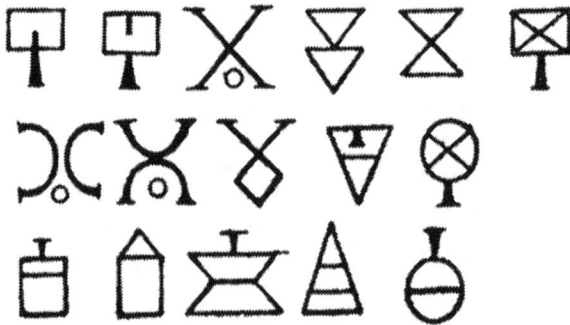

Saturno

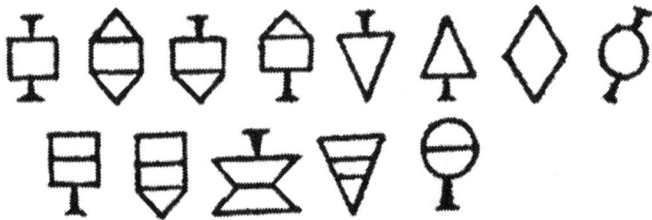

Dragón

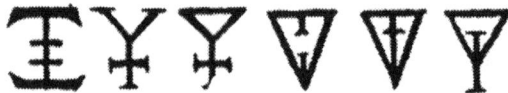

Dragón

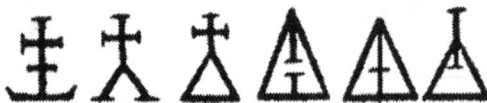

Tablas de Saturno

4	9	2
3	5	7
8	1	6

ד	ט	ב
ן	ה	ז
ח	א	ו

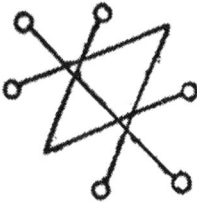

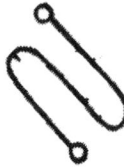

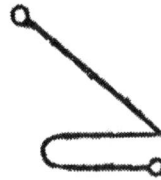

Tablas de Júpiter

4	14	15	1
9	7	6	12
5	11	10	8
16	2	3	13

ד	יה	יד	א
יצ	ז	ו	ט
ה	יא	י	ח
י	בכ	ג	יג

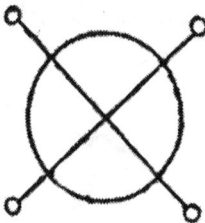

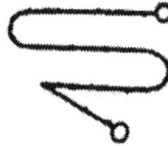

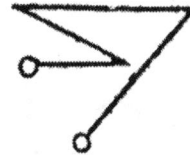

11 & 11aTables and Signs frequently used by Alchemists to bind planetary virtues and to effect Occultic healings in various disease processes. In every direction, the numbers added yield identical sum.

109

11a

Tablas de Marte

11	24	7	20	3
4	12	25	8	16
17	5	13	21	9
10	18	1	14	22
23	6	19	2	15

נ	כ	ז	כד	יא
יו	ח	כה	יב	ר
ט	כא	יג	ה	יד
כב	יד	א	יח	י
יה	כ	יט	ו	כו

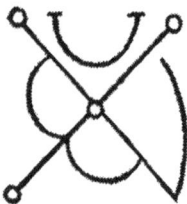
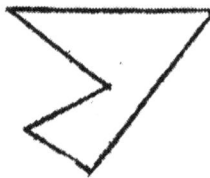
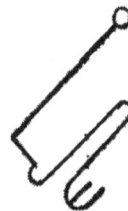

Tablas del Sol

6	32	3	34	35	1
7	11	27	28	8	30
19	14	16	15	23	24
18	20	22	21	17	13
25	29	10	9	26	12
36	5	33	4	2	31

א	לב	ג	לד	לה	ו
ז	חא	כז	כח	ח	ל
יט	יד	יו	ה	כג	כד
יח	כ	כב	כא	יז	יג
כה	כט	י	ט	כו	יב
לו	ה	לג	ד	ב	לא

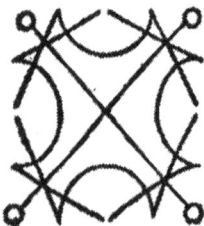
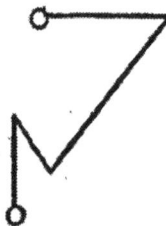
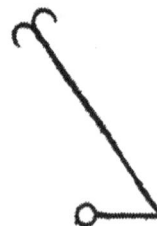

110

12

12, 12a & 12b Alchemical codes, celestial writings and Occult symbology through the ages. Hebrew, Greek, Latin and Kabbalistic letters and symbols were all used in the cryptic and mysterious records of the Medieval Alchemists and Paracelsian Occult Physicians to document the rare, exotic cures they effected on tumours, systemic infections, febrile conditions, veneral diseases and other varied illnesses of man.

12a

Teth, Jeth, Zain, Vav, Hei, Daleth, Guimel, Beth, Alef

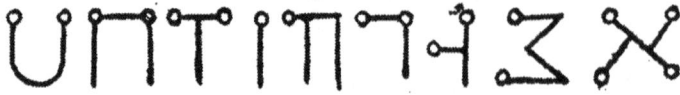

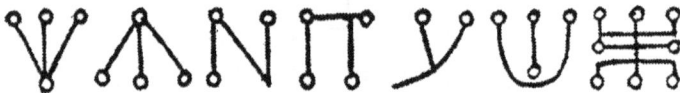

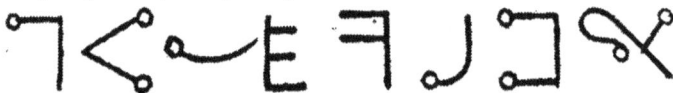

Tzadek, Pei, Eien, Samej, Nun, Mem, Lamed, Kuf, Iud,

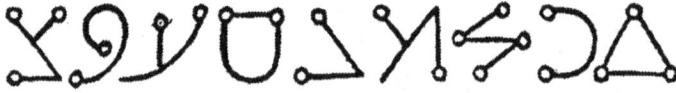

Thof, Shin, Reish, Kuf

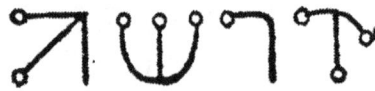

Zain, Vav, Hei, Daleth, Guimel, Beth, Alef

Nun, Mem, Lamed, Japh, Iud, Teth, Jeth,

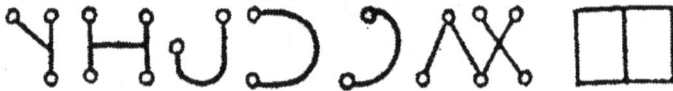

Reish, Kuf, Tzadek, Pei, Eien, Samej, Samej, Shin, Thof

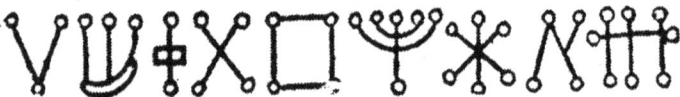

Jeth, Zain, Vav, Hei, Daleth, Guimel, Beth, Alef,

Samej, Nun, Mem, Lamed, Japh, Iud, Teth.

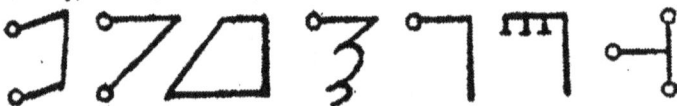

Thof, Shin, Reish, Kuf, Tzadek, Pei, Eien.

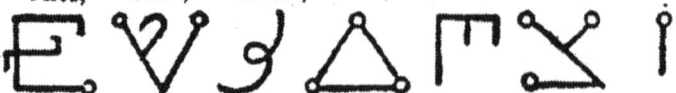

112

12b

113

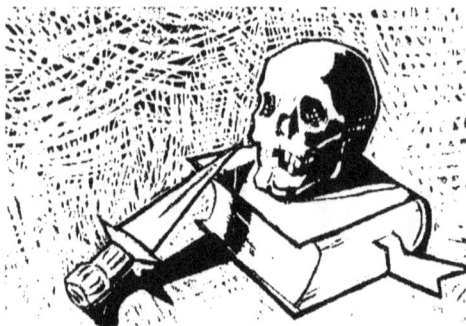

[13]Mystery of Initiation. Rites and Mystical ceremonies mark the Adept's admittance into the Higher studies of Ancient Esoteric Orders. The Alchemists were possessors of an exclusive gnosis that began in Egypt with the Pharaoh's Mystery Schools, and which survives today in the teachings of several Philosophical societies and Orders. The human skull, the ritualistic or ceremonial dagger and the *"Book of Splendours"* are part of the paraphernalia used in certain initiatory rituals of Occult Philosophy.

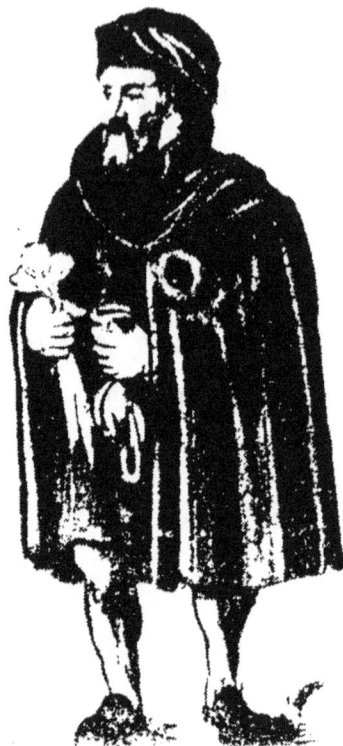

[14]Medieval Jewish Occult Physician. Noted for their profound knowledge of human anatomy and physiology, as well as their use of Occult methods in the treatment of a wide variety of life-treathening morbid conditions in man. They suffered bitter persecution under Medieval Christian kings and were victims of pogroms, exile and severe repressions.

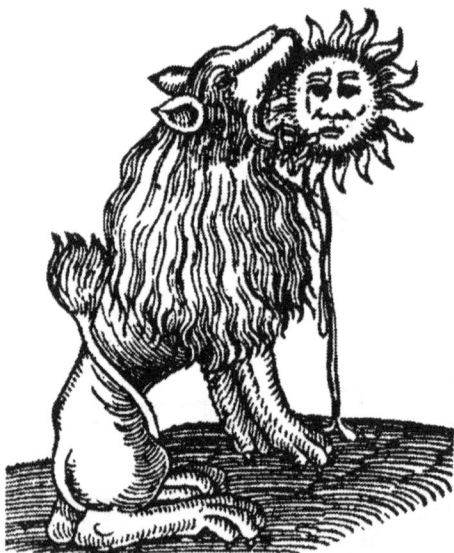

[15]The green lion devouring the Sun is an allegorical schema for a real chemical process in which aqua regia (nitric and hydrochloric acids) dissolved gold (the Sun). Because gold often carried copper impurities, the resulting liquid had a bluish-green tint, the lion's colour. (From a 16th century engraving).

114

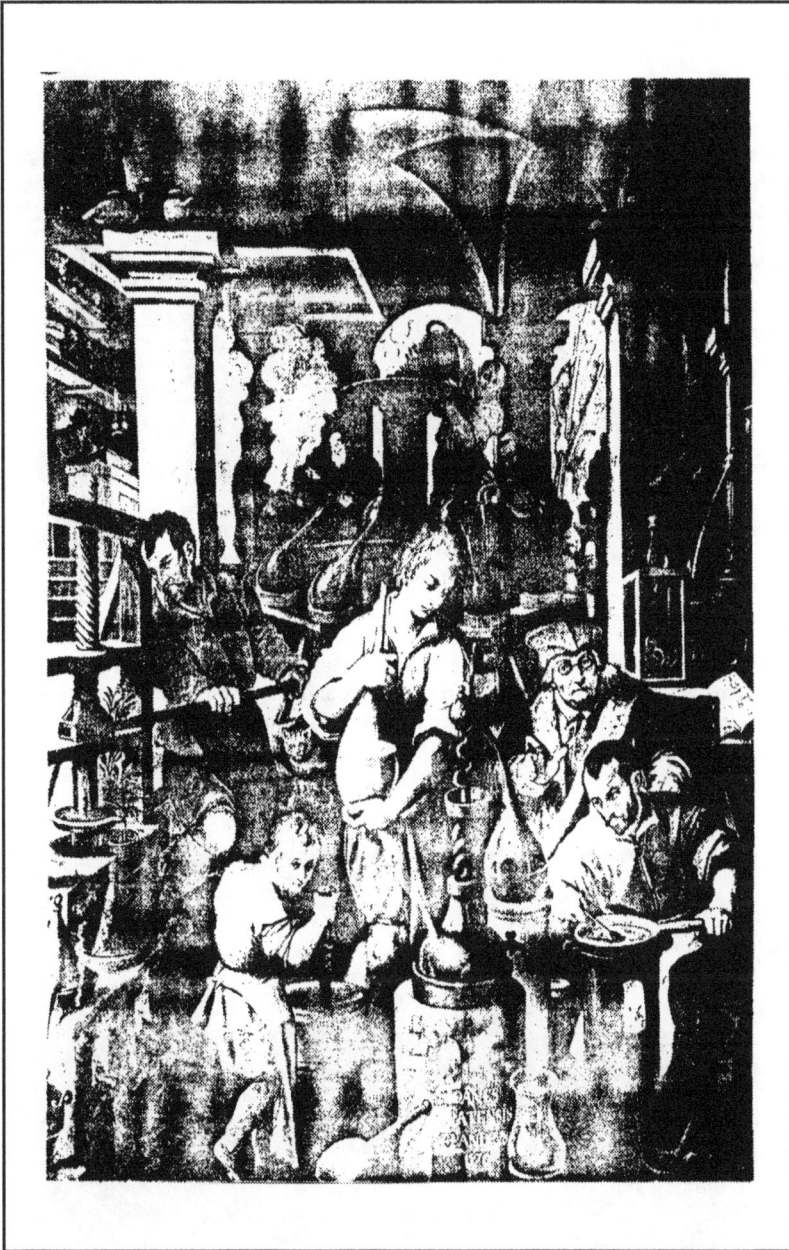

[16] 16th century alchemical laboratory. The alchemist points to the retort called the Philosopher's Egg, in which the magical gold-making substance known as the Philosopher's Stone would be formed. (From the works of Joanes Stratensis).

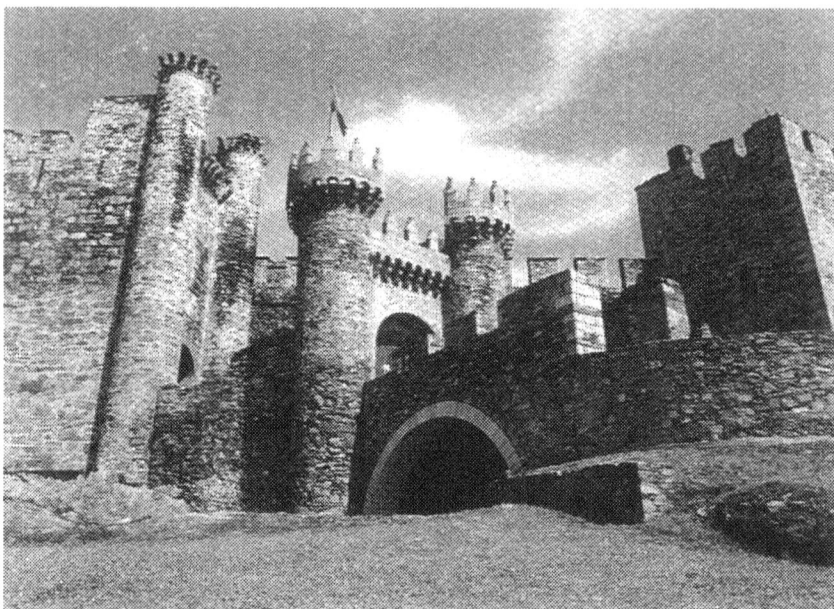

[17]Castle of the Knight Templars at Ponferrada, Spain. Was at one time the repository of an extensive collection of manuscripts, codices and books on Alchemy and Occult Medicine. Partly in ruins, it is now used for cultural and touristic purposes. (Courtesy: Junta de Castilla y León)

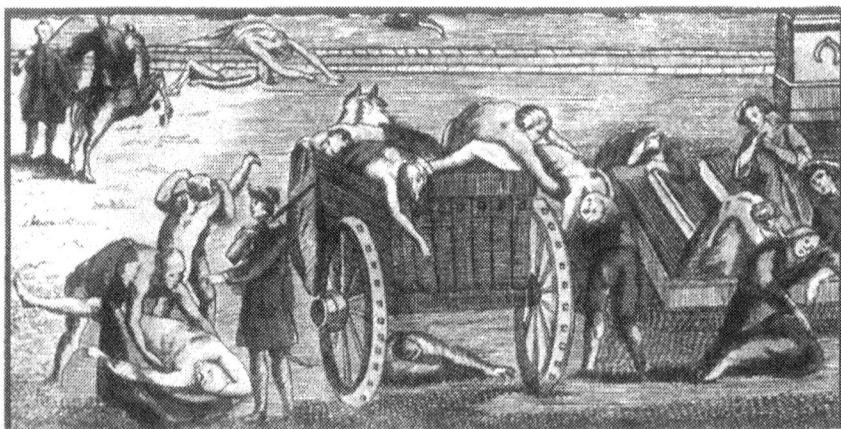

[18]The Plague (Black Death) in Marseilles, France. A XII century painting. (Courtesy:-Bibliothéque Nationale, Paris)

116

19a

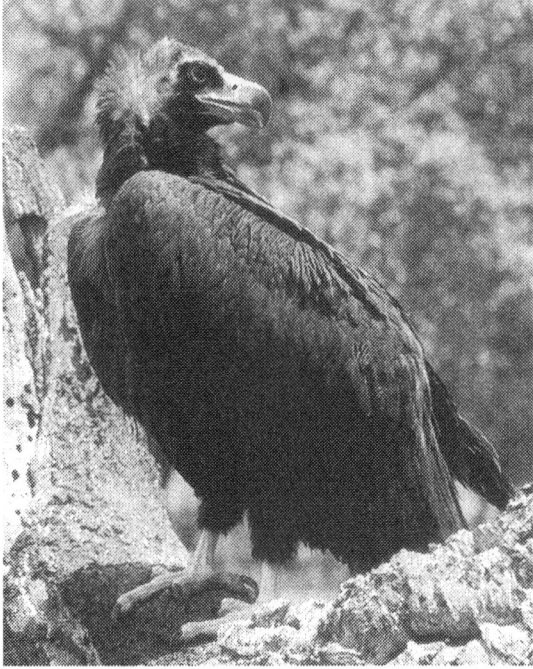

19b

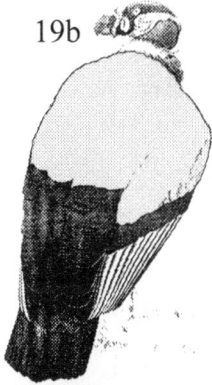

19d

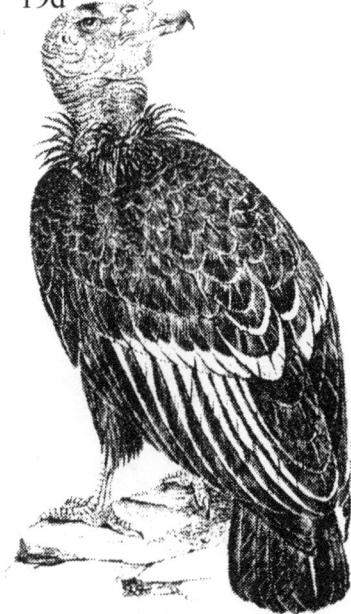

19c

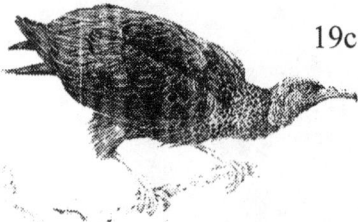

[19]Vultures, of the family 'Cathartidae" a) Black Vulture, b) King Vulture, c) California condor, d) Turkey vulture. Their immunity to diseases was noted by the Templars during the plague epidemic, the Black Death, in Medieval Europe.

117

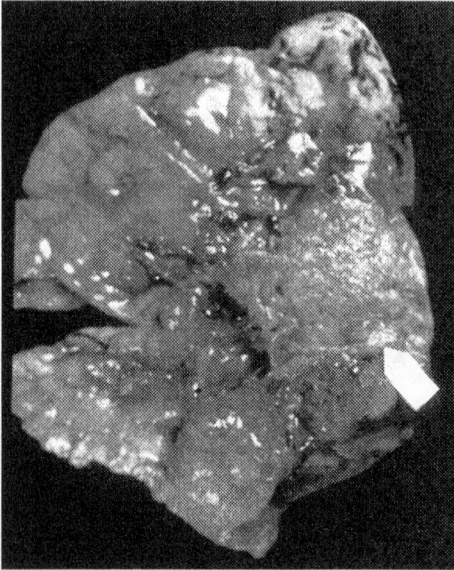
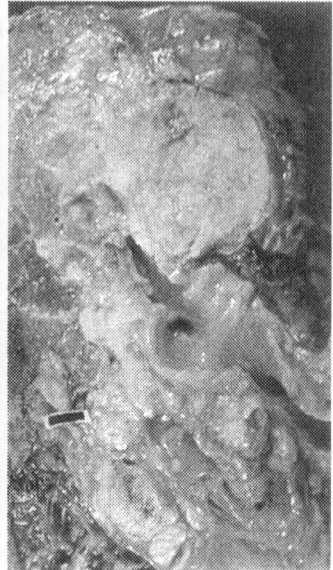

20x   20y

[20]Cancerous lung tissue (x and y) and inflammatory cancer of the breast.[z] (From the private papers of Dr. Héctor Valdés).

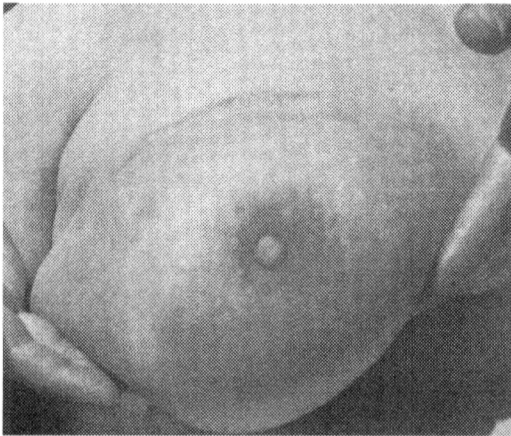

20z

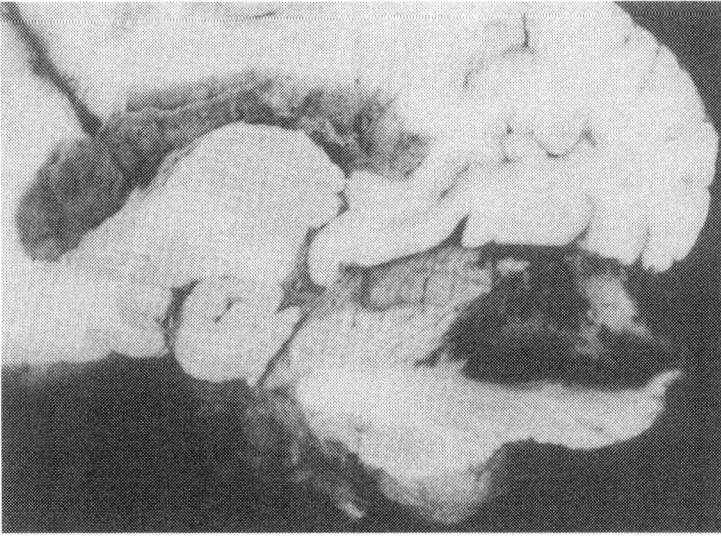

[21] A metastatic carcinoma of the cerebellum seen through centercut of the cerebral and cerebellar hemispheres. Cancerous tumour is dark sphere in lower right area of the superior surface of the cerebellum. The original tumour began as a bronchogenic carcinoma originating in the bronchus. (Private collection of Dr. Héctor Valdés).

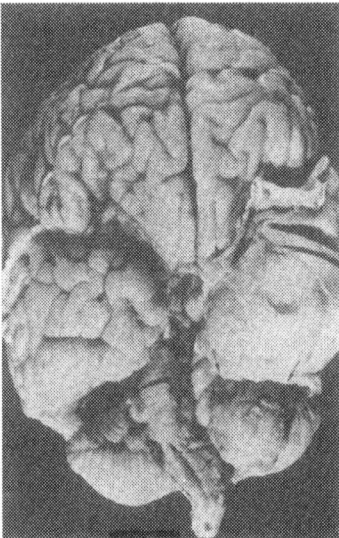

[22] A meningioma of the posterior area of base of the brain. It is an oval-shaped tumour mass (arrows) that has displaced the brain-stem, curving it to the opposite side. (Private collection of Dr. Héctor Valdés).

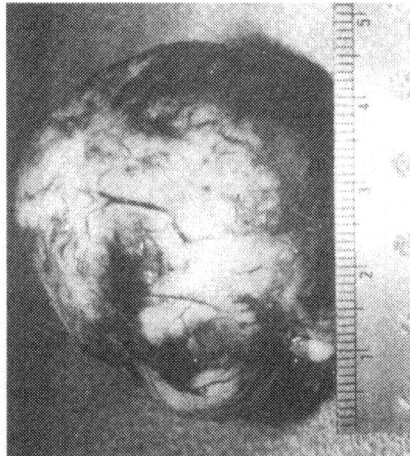

[23] This meningioma (slow growing tumour of the arachnoidal tissue) was removed from the area of the sphenoid bone – a large bone at base of skull, near outer aspect – Usually malignant and mostly seen in adults, it responded well to the Alchemical treatment as clinically confirmed by the Cisneros-Valdés team. (From the private papers of Dr. Héctor Velarde Valdés.)

119

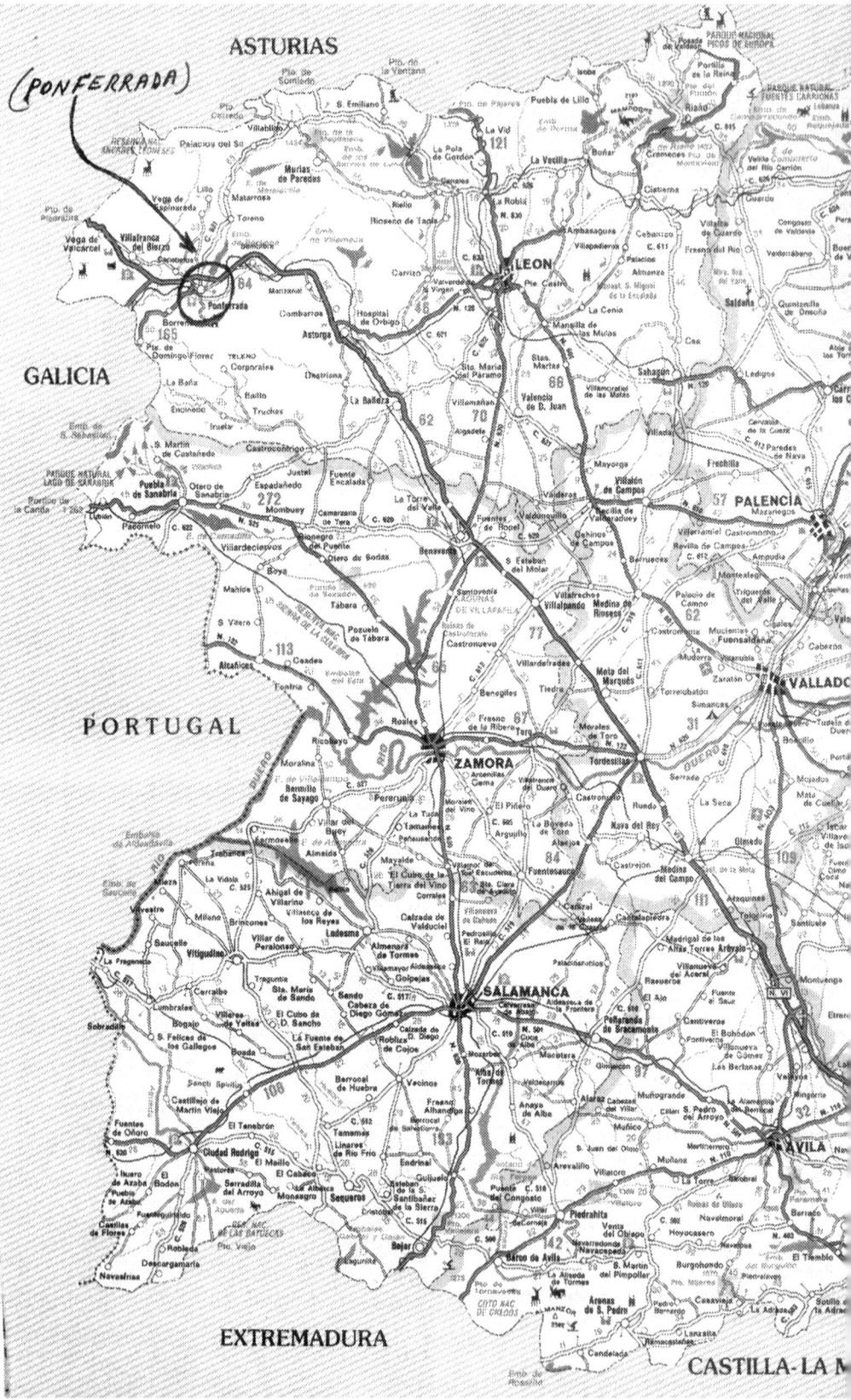

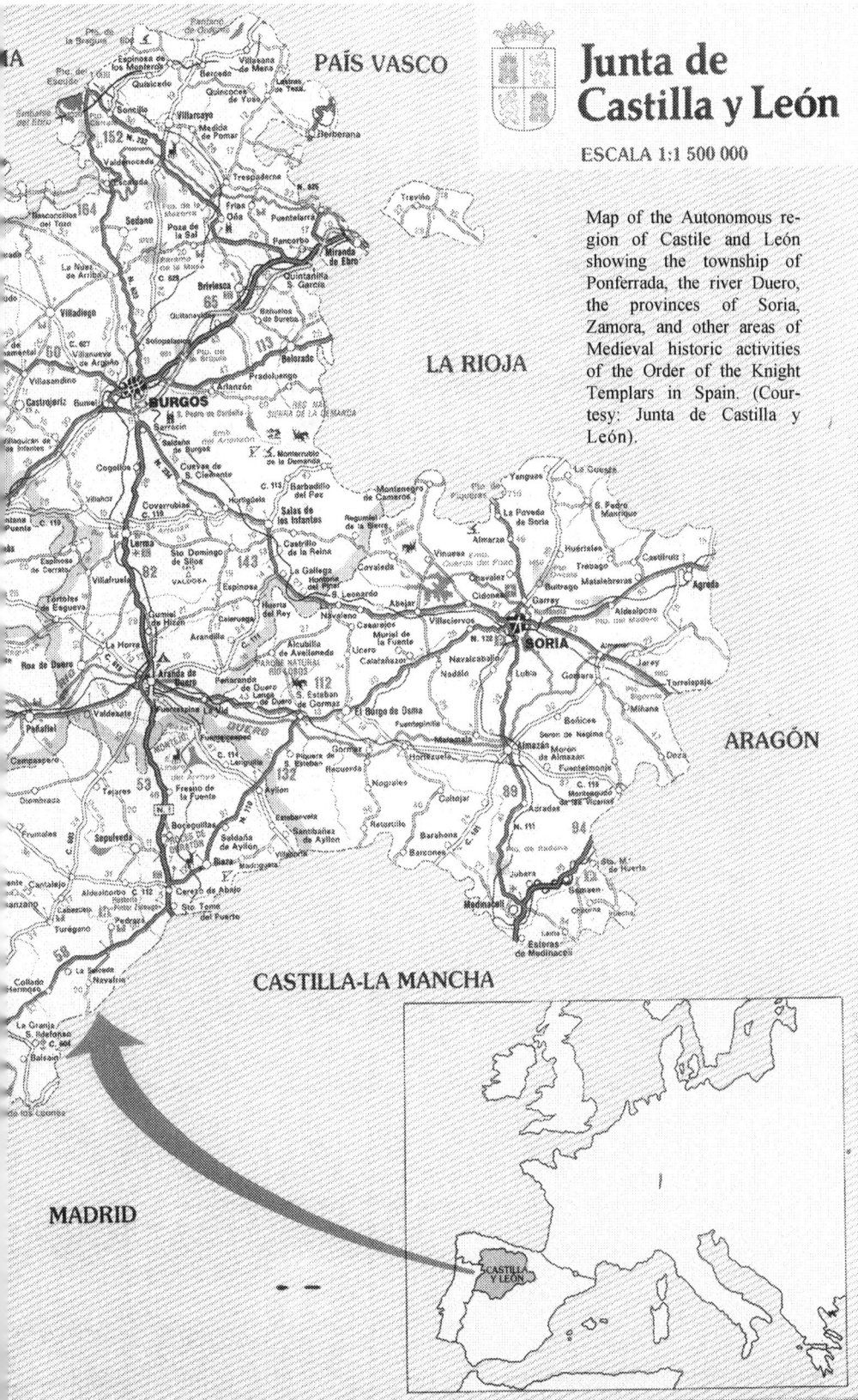

Junta de Castilla y León

ESCALA 1:1 500 000

Map of the Autonomous region of Castile and León showing the township of Ponferrada, the river Duero, the provinces of Soria, Zamora, and other areas of Medieval historic activities of the Order of the Knight Templars in Spain. (Courtesy: Junta de Castilla y León).

LA RIOJA

BURGOS

SORIA

ARAGÓN

CASTILLA-LA MANCHA

MADRID

CASTILLA Y LEÓN

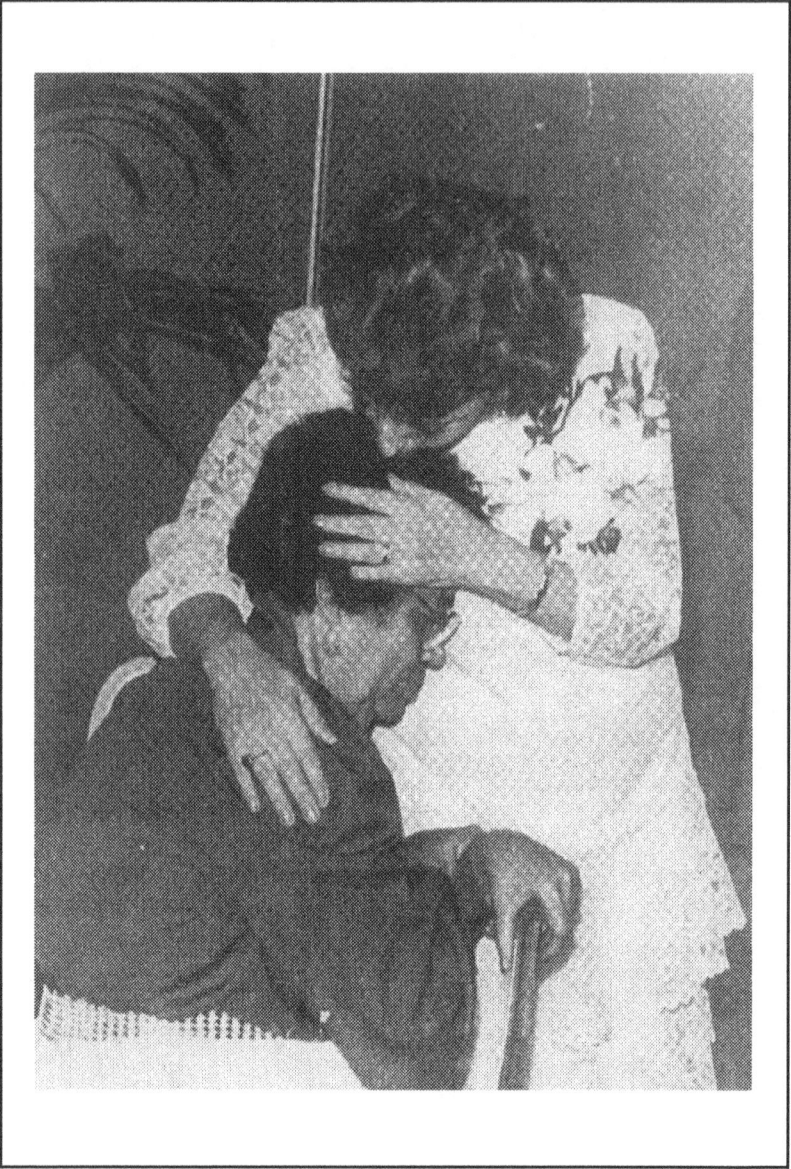

[24]A modern Oracle at work. Psychic visionary María Frasca attempts metaphysical cure during her eventful visit to Jamaica in 1989. Her prediction of the discovery of a cure for Cancer in Jamaica was met with great scepticism at the time. (*Daily Gleaner photo*).

Chapter 5

A Modern
Oracle Speaks

$\mathcal{I}$t was also during the notable decade of the 1980's that a series of mysterious events took place in Jamaica, with the emergence of Mrs. María Frasca, the Roman Catholic visionary from Florida who had accurately predicted, many months before, the island-nation's onslaught by tropical hurricanes "Allen" and later on in 1988, "Gilbert".

Mrs. Frasca, a mature, typical American white suburbanite, had for many years been experiencing frequent diurnal and nocturnal visions of the "Madonna", the perpetually virgin mother of Jesus Christ. As she vividly described the strange mystical phenomena, these came in the form of numerous visual and auricular apparitions of a dazzlingly beautiful lady radiating a luminous, extremely brilliant light.

The arresting and dramatic nature of the visions were frightening at first, but thereafter became so frequent – as many as three or four daily – that María Frasca quickly settled into a comfortable pattern of almost daily visionary episodes with the miraculous 'Queen of Heaven' and 'Mother of God'.

And this ethereal Lady would appear unto her almost anywhere and at any time, though more often at home; and she would usually, but not always, be cradling a small child in her arms. She was arrayed in either a sky-blue or white gown which also seemed to glow brightly; her feet were always enshrouded in a small dark cloud upon which she also appears to be standing.

The Madonna's facial expression was one of sweet kindness, mercy and genuine concern, exhuding an inescapable aura of saintly motherly love and sorrow for a 'wayward and sinful world'. And when the Virgin Mother spoke, in that mild, melodious and otherworldly voice that was so comforting and reasurring, the visionary felt within her innermost being, that she, a simple and ordinary housewife, albeit a devout Catholic, had for some unknown reason been favoured by a divine selection, to be the human conduit of momentous spiritual messages from the very heavenly sanctuary.

The supernatural visits would last at least five minutes, but often remain for up to twenty minutes, during which time other persons present in the same room or hall did not perceive the vision itself, but would definitely see evidence that María Frasca was obviously seeing and experiencing something which they were not. Yet, the inexplicable bright effulgence that invariably accompanied the vision, would be seen by all those present as a suspended orb of luminosity hovering at about two meters from the ground.

And these 'Virgin apparitions' were a profoundly disturbing epiphany for the pious devotee, proving to be irresistible to the senses; they were a series of noetic experiences during which she underwent an afflatus of the soul, with a variety of physical and mental effects persisting even through her routine of daily domestic activities. For, the Madonna displayed to María Frasca her spectacularly beautiful humanlike form, always surrounded by a radiating effulgence more luminous than the sun and personifying a fragmental manifestation of transcendental opulence that scintillates in all colours of the spectrum.

Not only was the visual impact of the miracle overwhelming to her perception, but the contents of the messages pronounced by the mythical being had so many astounding apocalyptic and prophetic features that were truly ominous, portentous and 'pregnant with doom', that she felt impelled to share those messages with the world, and especially with the people, church and governmental leaders unto whom the oracles were directed. And so she went about, diligently, with all the blind zealotry of her exacerbated cultic fanaticism. She became a harbinger of many woes and divers judgemental events of a catastrophic nature.

And when the Madonna spoke, deep felt stirrings of religious emotions would vibrate many responsive chords within María Frasca's long-conditioned mind. All the subtle, subliminal effects in symbol, colour, chant, incense and flame, along with the bewitching visual impact of pomp and pageantry of the Mass, had worked a marvellous receptiveness in her consciousness. Thus, in the Madonna visions she saw and heard that which from the early days of her catholic upbringing, she had been craftily prepared to behold.

Then the resplendently radiant Virgin Mother spoke unto the Seer, saying thus: "My child, I weep for humanity... My heart is filled with sorrow because of the unrepentant ones. Say unto them that the time of the end is near, and great disasters, unmitigated sufferings and all manner of major catastrophes shall befall the people if they do not repent and turn away from their sins."

"I stand ready to intercede with My son in heaven, and He shall accept My petitions on behalf of the lost ones, for I am His selfsame Mother, I... even I, who appeared also unto the faithful little ones at Lourdes, at Fatima and at Medjugorge[1]."

"Say also unto the people in the island of Jamaica, that they are very dear to the Madonna, and that land shall be a blessed land, for the heavens shall look upon her with favour. I am calling

---

[1] in Yugoslavia

the people of Jamaica to repentance and constant prayer, for great calamities shall befall them if they continue in their evil ways."

And so, in numerous subsequent visions, the heavenly apparition communicated many other messages to her worshipful devotee... Thereafter, Mrs. Frasca made it her paramount and unshakable duty, to deliver the extraterrestrial oracles and warnings to whomever will listen to her. Absolutely convinced of the divine character and origin of the celestial Lady, the psychic diligently transmitted the oracular warnings to Jamaica's Prime Minister during the course of lengthy telephone conversations from Florida. Among these were the uncannily accurate predictions on two devastating tropical hurricanes.

Numerous visionary episodes she experienced while in a state of trance of the ecstatic modality, during which her perception of reality was distorted and she remained entangled in a dense forest of delusion. And so, she went forth in the nescience of her idolatrous attachment, performing for the "Virgin" all the required acts of worship and faith that in passion and ignorance she eagerly carried out.

Her pilgrimage to the 'blessed land of Jamaica' was spurred by specific instructions given to her by the Madonna in one of the many visions she received in her home. The radiant being of light had said unto her: "There in Jamaica's Blue Mountains, by my instrumentality it shall be given unto you, land through which flows a stream of pure water... and besides those waters a holy shrine must be established to my name, and my consecrated statue shall be erected there. And those waters will become a healing balsam to all who suffer illness and in repentance turn to My Immaculate Heart for succour."

She arrived in the mystical island to a mixed reception from the largely fundamentalist Bible-loving Jamaicans; and certainly, a faithful Catholic citizen offered and gave to the visionary a portion of land in the rich coffee-growing Blue Mountain area, through which cascades a lively stream of crystalline spring water, But, that brief sojourn in the tropical paradise turned out to be a turbulent one for the matronly American psychic, and the Blessed

Virgin seemed unable to turn events in her favour... for now at least.

****

Josefina de Cisneros had been placed under that condition of semi-trance known as 'Twilight Sleep', a form of partial anaesthesia, or subconsciousness, which dulls awareness to pain. It also softens or effaces memory of pain, such as that of childbirth. It is produced by hypodermic injection of Morphine and Scopolamine, the latter being an alkaloid obtained from the roots of the plant Scopolia of the nightshade family.

Her physician had administered the narcotic to alleviate the severe undulating pain and acute depression she was undergoing as a result of her recent miscarriage. The experience had been a devastating one for her, as this was her first pregnancy, and both, herself and her husband were excitedly looking forward to the advent of their first child with much hope and boundless joy.

As she slowly emerged from the drowsiness and dream-like state induced by the narcoleptic drugs, a multitude of confusing thoughts paraded by on the screen of her consciousness, seemingly beyond the control of her will. While silently mourning the loss of her baby, she bravely fought off the negative depressive mood that frequently threatened to overcome her, and by the sheer force of a rigorous mental refocusing, managed to cogitate instead on her immediate future and the many challenging tasks awaiting her.

After seven weeks of convalescence, and having obviously recuperated from most of the physical, though not psychological ravages brought about by the painful loss, she had to return to the university to sit for an oral defense of her doctoral thesis. She considered herself fortunate to have been accepted at the prestigious University of Salamanca. Established in 1218, it is the oldest in Spain and one of the finest in Europe. Although at the dawn of the 19th century it suffered considerable damage during the Napoleonic wars, it later recovered and enjoyed a great revival which restored its worldwide fame and reputation.

She was often awestruck at the majestic and imposing façade of the university, which has a central circular medallion standing out among the profuse ornamentation typical of the Plateresque style. That medallion has an effigy of the Catholic King and Queen and above it there is the coat of arms of Emperor Carlos V.

In spite of the gruelling four hour long session before a panel of eminent academicians, Josefina felt strangely relieved and elated. It had been over five years of relentless hard work punctuated by very difficult research assignments, and field and study projects. Her thesis advisor and mentor at the Faculty of Philosophy had been greatly impressed by her methodical and profoundly analytical philosophical essays, and did not hesitate in recommending her for the task of compiling a comprehensive history of the Order of the Knight Templars that was commissioned by the provincial Masonic Lodge.

And so it was, that two weeks later, armed with an introductory letter from the illustrious Grand Master of the lodge, Josefina and her husband left Salamanca and headed towards the small township of Ponferrada in the province of León in northwest Spain, not far from the border with Portugal. They were on a curious mission, hoping to gain access to valuable information contained in a rare private collection of ancient manuscripts that were rumoured to be deposited at one of the many old castles still in the area.

The Spanish province of León had always been subjected to invasions by many peoples and nations, and throughout its history has seen the land occupied by Barbarians, Arabs, Mozarabs, the French and the Romans, among others. In 68 AD the Seventh Roman Legion, Gemina Pia Felix, set up camp and gave birth to the city of León, seat of the provincial administration.

While on their exotic quest for the reputed ancient collection of Alchemical and historical records, they could not escape the quaint charm and historic legacy of the region with it numerous monuments, chapels, pantheon, museums, archives and palaces, all mute testimonials to the former glories and rich cultural heritage of the Spanish empire.

They had arrived in Ponferrada just when the religious festival of 'La Encina' was taking place, with its colorful processions through the town's narrow streets, traditional dances, displays of typical articles and the sampling of local products. Their gastronomic fancies were titillated by a variety of regional delicacies such as trout soup, wild boar, frogs legs, El Bierzo-style octopus, 'botillos' (stuffed pig's stomach) and of course, the excellent wines and brandies of the region.

Two days later they motored on to nearby Villafranca del Bierzo, a noble, refined and artistic town, where they seeked out and found the coffered church of San Francisco. The introductory letter in their possession was addressed to the local priest there. He in turn, took the visitors to Astorga, another provincial township where they had audience with the Bishop at his ornate and luxurious centuries-old palace.

Dr. Cisneros and his wife were allowed to visit the Castle of Ponferrada accompanied by the priest and a curator from the Benedictine Mother's Museum. No item was to be removed from the Castle, but they could freely photograph or copy any document from the extensive collection of old manuscripts, codices, maps and various historical records kept there.

And the five hundred year old castle of Ponferrada proved to be an unparalleled repository of rare medieval treasures and artistic relics, all of which were carefully housed throughout its numerous vaults, galleries, towers and armoury.

The Grand Master had promised to provide Profesora Cisneros with authentic research material she could source, in order to properly document her work. Sometime after, he informed her that she would be allowed almost unrestricted access to the extensive library of Occult and Esoteric writings kept at the feudal Castle of Ponferrada. This was an imposing and highly complex military fortress and one of the largest castles in northwest Spain. It was constructed in the Middle Ages and built over a period of two centuries, from the 13th to the 15th, and *belonged to the Order of the Knight Templars.* Composed of a large polygonal bailey with double and triple defences forming barbicans, watchtowers, living quarters and a large courtyard, it also had many underground passages, dungeons, and several tunnels connecting the Castle to nearby churches, monastic cloisters and convents. These secret underpass have all been sealed-off in recent times.

And, this impressive Castle of Ponferrada, was merely one of many such heavily fortified structures which the secretive Templars had erected throughout most of western Europe. The Order of the Knight Templars was a religious and military order established with papal blessing about 1118 AD at Jerusalem, for the express purpose of protecting pilgrims to the Holy Land, and safeguarding the Holy Sepulcher. For a time they had occupied quarters next to the remains of Solomon's Temple.

The highly disciplined and militant Order of 'pious soldiers' had rapidly extended its influence among the aristocracy and nobility of France, Belgium, Spain, Portugal and Germany, with an especially strong presence in Italy's papal court. Their growing control of international banking and finance made the order particularly powerful, to the extent that they were, for a time at least, the 'de facto' bankers to the Popes, and money lenders to many Kings.

The hierarchy of the Order's leadership came from the nobles and aristocrats of the countries in which the Order was openly active; they nevertheless maintained secret agents in virtually every important nation of Medieval Europe where they were covertly involved in the many complex international intrigues of the times. Their presence in Crusader Jerusalem during the 12th and 13th centuries, came about mainly as a result of their ages-old quest for the Biblical Ark of the Covenant, a relentless search that took them to the land of Ethiopia in the days of King Lalibella. They are reputed to have been the mysterious master builders of that East African kingdom's famous monolithic churches which were entirely carved out of rock monolith, employing a still unknown laser-like technology to etch out intricate inner and outer details in the profusely ornate churches. These also are connected by secret underground tunnels and passages.

The extensive international network of Templar castles, palaces, monasteries and various cloisters, greatly facilitated the constant traffic from many countries which saw the officials of the Order going to and fro all over Europe, the Near and Middle East and North Africa. Within the Spanish Autonomy of Castile and León, there was a special correspondence and inter-provincial travel of Templar brethren, from the Castle of Ponferrada at the Western limits of the region, right across to its Eastern border in the province of Soria where the placid and navigable river Duero is born, crossing the land of fine green pines and villages both old and noble.

The first reference to its capital, Soria, is from 868 AD when its inhabitants rose up against the usurping ruler, the Emir of Córdoba. Conquered and repopulated in the 11th and 12th centuries, it became part of the Kingdom of Castile in 1136. Alfonso VIII rewarded the faithfulness of Soria with many privileges, and Alfonso X conceded it the status of a city. It was during the Middle Ages that the province was divided into districts, giving rise to the *twelve linages,* a unique, hereditary institution from which all the nobles in Soria have descended.

The 'twelve linages' of aristocratic Castilian nobility was originally conceived by Templar adherents for the purpose of ensuring a continuity of the organization's long-term trans-generational aims of world hegemony, while at the same time keeping the upper ranks of the Order's hierarchy within the firm grip of the descendants of the blood-connected nobility. From this time henceforth, the designation 'Don' (De Origen Noble / of Noble Birth) prefixed the family names of the titled aristocracy in Spain.

It is there, on the left bank of the river Duero in the outskirts of Soria, that the Romanesque-style, old Templar Monastery of San Juan de Duero is located, still containing the colonnade of its extremely unusual cloisters. The river Duero served as a connecting river 'highway' between the Templar Monastery and the Castle at Ponferrada, and on many occasions throughout the turbulent history of the region, entire libraries of manuscripts and precious relics and even fleeing aristocrats out of favour with officialdom, would be given sanctuary and protection at one or the other Templar center.

The hundreds of miles of scenic countryside through which the historic river flows, were easily navigated in barges and river boats from Soria to the western province of Zamora, from where they would transfer to smaller tender that would easily negotiate the winding smaller rivers and lakes right up to a point near to Ponferrada. The Duero's watery course traverses five provinces from Soria to León, and along the way a series of strategically located sanctuaries, convents, monasteries and churches provided convenient resting places for the taciturn and morose Templars on their baleful pursuits.

After two weeks of diligent search of the old archives at the Castle, the Cisneros' duo came across a startling revelation that was not only surprising and thoroughly shocking, but one that seemed to have been unknown outside of the furtive organization. To Dr. Axel Cisneros, the quaint old Spanish manuscripts, replete with the obscure symbology typical of Medieval Alchemy, unequivocally documented what could easily be one of the earliest experiments on morbid pathology ever carried out.

It was around the year 1347, after the devastating plague had ravaged Asia, that the much feared pestilence appeared in the Crimea where the infected Mongol hordes of invaders were besieging the fortified Genoese trading post of Kaffa (now Feodosiya). As reported by Templar agents to their superiors, the invaders had called off their attack after the mysterious disease swiftly reduced their numbers, but before withdrawing they delivered a deadly parting shot. Using giant-sized catapults, they hurled the still-warm bodies of their own plague victims over the city walls, spreading the deadly infection within the enclosed settlement, in what was perhaps one of the earliest instances of germ warfare on record.

Some of the Genoese defenders managed to escape and boarded their galleys leaving the plague-ridden port. As they sailed on, the pestilence spread to every port they visited, and in a matter of months the whole of Europe was thoroughly in the grips of the deadliest pandemic in the history of mankind, a truly brutal demographic catastrophe of biblical proportions, for in less than two years, more than one third of Europe's population, or about 25 million persons, perished, as the terrible disease swept through the unsanitary hovels of the continent. The whole of Europe was riddled with death as the grim reaper covered Spain, England, Italy, France, Scandinavia, Germany, Austria, Switzerland and the Baltics, to leap even across the Mediterranean to North Africa.

Medieval Europe was then in the stranglehold of pervasive religious superstitions; women began using lipstick to discourage demons from entering a woman's mouth and possessing her, and covering the mouth while yawning arose from the notion that one's soul could escape through a wide-open mouth. The Black Death was also viewed as a form of Divine Judgement, a punishment from God himself. Consequently, in the midst of the widespread panic among the population, Pope Clement VI declared the year 1350 to be a Holy Year, causing thousands of pilgrims to visit Rome as they had been promised direct access to paradise without having to pass through purgatory. The hundreds of thousands of pilgrims who heeded the call, spread the disease as they travelled, across the breadth and length of the plague-racked continent.

The personal physician of Pope Clement VI, Guy de Chauliac, who was also a high Templar official, had graphically described the two types of plague that had invaded Europe: pneumonic and bubonic. This they saw in a secret report he had sent to his superiors in the Order, and which read in part: "The first (pneumonic) lasted two months, with continuous fever and spitting of blood, and from this, one died in three days. The second (bubonic) lasted for the rest of the period, with continuous fever but also with apostumes (abscesses) and carbuncles on the external parts, principally on the armpits and groin. From this, one died in five days."

As no one knew how the disease was transmitted, efforts to control the epidemic were in vain, though many suspected that contact with a sufferer, or his clothing, was dangerous. In Florence, Italy, residents blamed the plague on its cats and dogs and proceeded to slaughter these animals, unaware that in so doing they were freeing the creature actually involved in spreading the contamination, the rat. But the church benefited greatly from the deadly plague, for men and women gave all they had to the church, hoping that God would protect them from illness. Enormous wealth poured into the coffers of the church and all manner of lucky charms, images of Christ and the saints, perfumes, vinegar and special potions were said to ward off the disease.

An epidemic of plague in human beings is usually preceded by an epizootic of rats, the rat being the common animal vector of this disease. Infected fleas migrate to man from dying or dead rats and, while feeding, deposit infected material (dejecta or regurgitated blood), in or on the skin. The pneumonic form of plague, however, can be transmitted from man to man by droplet infection, and may appear during the height of an epidemic.

From their point of entry the infecting organisms spread throughout the body via lymph channels and the blood stream. Regional lymph nodes become swollen and packed with leukocytes. Spread to other organs often is extensive, producing foci of suppuration and necrosis (death of areas of tissue or bone) in the liver, lungs, spleen and brain. The pneumonic form is rapidly fatal. "Petechiae", the black spots that give the disease the name "black death" may appear about the third day.

And while the horrendous epidemic wreaked its grim toll upon the helpless European population, the monastic cloisters had drastically curtailed all contact with the outside world, and the heavily garbed monks only ventured out under force of dire necessity. The Order of the Knight Templars had by then decided to embark on a curious experimental observation of the course of the plague disease, and in a series of carefully designed procedures were able to arrive at surprising conclusions, all of which were meticulously recorded and kept at the Castle of Ponferrada.

******

The Cisneros husband-wife team did not immediately attempt to read or interpret the many inscribed texts they saw in the fragile, decaying pages of those musty records. They saw therein detailed drawings of enormous trap cages that were built with sturdy tree branches tied together with vines at the corners. Then, strewn on the ground within the cages were what appeared to be portions of partially eaten human cadavers upon which several huge vulture-like birds were perched. Numerous descriptive notes and enigmatic symbols were seen profusely surrounding the central drawings, some of which were faded and barely discernible.

From these preliminary observations they had concluded that the laboriously inscribed and richly ornate notations, most of which appeared to be in Classical Latin, merely elaborated upon that which the skillfully drawn illustrations effectively portrayed: huge carrion-eating birds feeding on the bodies of plague victims within those house-sized caged enclosures. Some distance away, the enshrouded figures of several monks could be seen and at the extreme corner of the lower section of the picture, a trenchlike mass grave, a veritable 'plague pit' replete with corpses, completed the grim portrayal of that medieval 'experiment'.

Dr. Cisneros' wife wondered aloud that even the characteristic 'petechiae' or black spots of plague-ridden bodies could easily be discerned on these diseased 'tenements of clay' shown in the quaintly-drawn pictures. But, it was Axel Cisneros who called his wife's attention to a curious detail in those illustrations which had seemingly leapt at his eyes. Several of the vultures had what appeared to be 'beards', the unmistakable identifying feature of the 'Lammergeyer' (Gypaetus Barbatus), the largest European bird of prey which inhabits the lofty mountains of Southern Europe, Asia and North Africa.

These huge raptorial birds have a very large wingspan (up to 3 metres) and 'vibrissa', the dark beardlike feathers on either side of its beak. They also saw there, other types of vultures in those drawings... among them the Turkey Vulture and the Black Vulture.

They both marvelled at the fact that up to this day, in the deep ravines that the river Duero has cut into the lands of Sayago in the Spanish province of Zamora, there is an area known as "Los Arribes" which is the protected habitat of a wide variety of birds of prey. And in the nearby province of Segovia, in the same autonomous region of Castile and León, there is the Riaza gorge, a sheer limestone canyon which even now is colonized by one of the largest reserves of the bearded vulture, the Lammergeyer, in all Europe. This was the selfsame geographical area of activity of the Templars some 600 years ago.

Weeks later, they had returned to Salamanca with a vast cache of photographic material obtained at the Castle of Ponferrada. These were enlarged after careful processing, and when scrutinized and compared to other historical records in Josefina's possession, the Cisneros couple realized that they had just acquired a most extraordinary ancient record, giving detailed descriptions of a series of crude and basic experimental observations carried out during the Middle Ages in Europe by the Order of the Knight Templars, into the origin and causes of certain disease processes.

It was Professor Josefina Velarde de Cisneros who translated most of the material from Latin to Spanish, and who also interpreted the ubiquitous Alchemical and Occult symbology for her husband. And so it was, that the Knight Templars who were in Ponferrada, Spain, up to the 14th century, had been keen and meticulous scientific observers and innovators of no mean order.

Each of those ancient folios containing either text or illustrations of this notable episode in the Templars historic experimental study of the Black Death contagion, were headed by the Occult symbol of the 'Lamniscate'. Resembling a horizontalized numeral 8(∞) and signifying 'infinity' in the mundane sciences, the Lamniscate is really a very ancient Alchemical symbol constructed by the joining of two sine curves. It was used by the Alchemists to depict the "Schema of the Elements of Alchemy" which was the centerpiece of Occult Medicine's principle of the Cyclic Thermal variations that regulate all living organisms. According to Paracelsus, it represents the flux of biological cycles... the so-called "four modes of the vital life force" which must be kept in equilibrium for optimal health.

In the ancient study of human physiology based on the principles of Occult Medicine, there is a postulate that says, "there is a *qualitative connection* between the types of desires, types of emotions, and modes of perception dominating an individual's personality." These patterns of our sensory mechanisms are integrated into the Alchemical concept of human temperamental types or classes.

The millennial Khamitic philosophy of ancient Egypt outlined the *Spiritual Anatomy* of man in their cosmogonical system known as the *Tree of Life,* establishing there that one of the basic biological forces in man is the Thermal (heat or fiery) factor that determines the level of biochemical activities in our bodies. The other basic force is the Hydration (water) factor which represents the universal medium in which all living things dwell.

It is well known that the life dwelling in each cell making up living beings, actually lives in water. Thus, the upper and the lower boundaries of this Thermal factor in living beings are relatively denoted as "Hot" and "Cold", while the upper and lower boundaries of the Hydration factor of bodies are denoted as "Moist" and "Dry". All biological activities can be reduced and explained by these two modalities, which is also the basis of traditional Chinese medical theory. The interaction of these two factors (Thermal and Hydration, or Fire and Water) produces the four modalities underlying all manifestations in the world. They have been symbolized as *The Four Elements of Alchemy.*

As understood by the ancient Alchemists, water is cold and moist, and it accumulates in bodies as they cool down. Then, as bodies begin to heat up, and have not yet lost their humidity, they are metaphorized as "air" (hot and moist). When the temperature rises to the upper ranges and bodies lose their humidity, they are metaphorized as "fire" (hot and dry). Finally, when they begin

Schema of the Elements of Alchemy
(From The Tree of Life, Cosmogonical System)

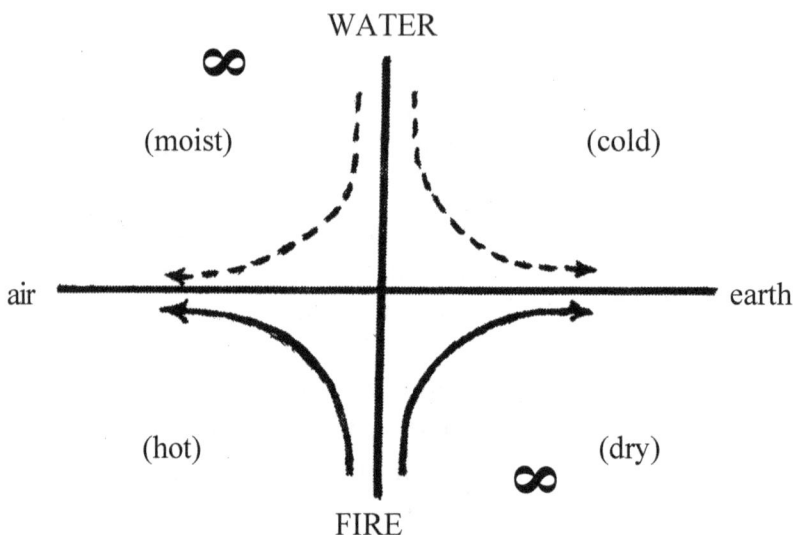

to cool down, but have not yet regained their moisture, they are metaphorized as "earth" (cold and dry).

It must be noted that all bodies go through these changes daily *with the rise and fall of temperature that follows the sun.* Therefore, in Occult Medicine, humans are classified as illustrated in the Alchemical Schema, as: "Fiery", "Watery", "Earthy" and "Airy". These are metaphors for the various types of human beings *according to their metabolic differences.* So then, "Fiery" people are "hot and dry", that is, they are of a *high catabolic activity,* which places their body-heat in the higher ranges, thereby increasing the rate of their physical and psychological activities. They are also lively, impatient, easy to anger, zealous and prone to acute illnesses. "Watery" people are the opposite, being "cold and moist".

These differences in the rate of metabolic activity in humans, and which are caused by bodily thermal variations, are of fundamental importance to the anti-tumour action of the ZAM-2RO biological compound. An analogy of this mechanism of thermal changes takes place in the life-sap of plants and in the humours or body fluids of animals. This rhythmic, solar-coordinated thermal oscillation is more pronounced or intense in certain species of plants and animals, being the "virtues" so well-known to all Occultists and Alchemists.

******

The serfs and local peasantry dwelling in the surrounding countryside at Ponferrada would daily see the dark and somber silhouettes of the monks in profile against the early morning sunrise, as they quietly and methodically walk up and down the high battlements of the fortified Knight Templars castle.

As they held their watchtower lookout duties, eagerly trying to get a glimpse of their brethren approaching in the misty distance, the devastating plague pandemic seemed so far away and remote to the solitude and quiet of their safe enclave. The expected emissaries would bring news from the sites of their secretive experiments with the vultures...

For, when the caged carrion-eaters were fed the corpses of Black Death victims and that of others who had died of the "Wasting Disease" (proliferative tumours), the designated purpose was to observe under controlled conditions, an anticipated pathological manifestation of the disease in the baleful birds.

And indeed, their crude experimentation was aimed at determining whether or not the vultures would survive the then unknown 'potent contaminating factor' in the fulminating plague pandemic, the Black Death that was rapidly decimating the helpless population. By means of the enormous trap-cages, they ensured the vultures' exclusive consumption of the diseased human flesh.

Some two centuries after the Knight Templars had left their castle in Ponferrada, the Master Alchemist and Occult Physician Cornelius Agrippa developed the secret Alchemical cure for proliferative tumours (Cancer) based on the experimental observations carried out on the corpses of Black Death victims by those militant warrior-monks in Medieval Spain.

He already knew that the carrion-eating vultures are virtually immune to every and all disease processes, and that these despised birds die only due to old age or traumatic injury. For, the Templars curious 'controlled study' had merely confirmed the fact that there is *a particular virtue* disseminated throughout the vulture's body, which gives it that absolute immunity to all diseases, and allows it to consume all manner of putrid, rotten and diseased tissues of any kind, with no possibility of being adversely or detrimentally affected by it.

And it was not only Agrippa, but also many other notable Alchemists and Occult Physicians, who had conducted detailed, profound studies of these wrongly maligned birds, so as to ascertain the precise locus of their marvellous protective virtue. Once this was determined, ways would be found to effect a transfer of the active anti-disease factor (or virtue) unto sick humans.

It was known in Medieval Europe that vultures were held to be sacred birds in ancient Egypt, and even though these soaring large birds of prey are closely related to hawks and eagles, significant differences set them apart. The Black vulture is a scavenger and eats dead animals almost exclusively. Its bald head allows him to keep his neck from becoming too filthy when it sticks its head into a carcass. Due to daily contact with dead animals, the vulture was wrongly assumed to have no sense of smell, however, early experiments have shown that it does have a keen sense of smell, for they are able to detect dead animals from great distances in the air though the animals were covered up to prevent them being seen.

Their characteristic graceful flight is due to the fact that they soar on rising thermal currents of air, and they eat not only carrion but also excrement and sometimes even garbage. The bill of a vulture is hooked and powerful, which it uses to tear the flesh off the bones of carcasses, and surely, it prefers to wait patiently for days even, until a dead animal begins to decay, before eating the flesh.

And by the time that Cornelius Agrippa left the Royal Courts of the King of Spain to take refuge with the French Burgundian monarchs, he had already concluded, and correctly so, that the concentrated source of the vultures universal immunity to diseases was *in its Gastric juices,* from whence it was further disseminated into the blood of the loathsome bird of prey.

Agrippa had drawn extensively from the writings of Claudius Galen, the noted Greek physician and medical writer (c. 130-200 AD) residing in Rome, where he was personal physician to Emperor Marcus Aurelius. And in the private writings of Galen, a pointed and persistent interest into the natural history, anatomy, physiology, reproduction and habitat of the Black and the Turkey vultures is most evident. For, Galen certainly alluded to certain curative qualities exhibited by humours (or fluids) that were obtained from this species of scavenging birds. Other esoteric writings reveal that in ancient Egypt the ovum of vultures was regarded as most precious, being used by the priests-physicians of those days as the principal ingredient in many potent therapeutics and medical potions.

And this digestive juice of the gastric glands of the stomach of vultures has many remarkable virtues or qualities, for, apart from being strongly acidic and containing various inorganic salts, it also has the intrinsic factor of the antianemic principle. Then, the mixture of its acid with several enzymes also present in the gastric juice has effects that neither substance has alone, and acts upon putrid, diseased tissues with truly surprising speed.

Cornelius Agrippa, like other medieval Alchemists and Occult Physicians had succeeded in developing their secret cure for proliferative tumours (Cancer) and many other intractable and intercurrent diseases, by combining specific galenicals (herbs and vegetable medicines) with *a concentrated extract derived from the gastric juice of vultures.*

******

"María Frasca has been an established and gifted psychic for many years. Through meditation she is able to realise indications of the future, both positive and negative... Mrs. Frasca's predictions for next year are..." and the local Jamaican newspaper, The Daily Gleaner, goes on to enumerate a number of frightening events usually of a catastrophic nature, that would befall the beautiful island of Jamaica and its people, if they do not repent and heed the timely warnings of the Madonna, the 'Mother of God'.

She had returned to the tropical, gemlike isle of the Caribbean, where an astute and well-designed media campaign had prepared her devotees and others, to throng the many meetings, seminars and press conferences that were organized for her visit. And again she did come armed with an abundance of portentous sayings that were pregnant with doom, eager as she was, to instill fear and trembling in the hearts of the natives, whom they had once called a despicable and noxious race of troglodytes, coarse and uncouth.

And many messages she claimed to have received in visions of the Madonna; these being in the form of specific instructions that she felt compelled to carry out. A beautiful statue of the Virgin Mary had been commissioned to skilled Italian sculptors and was already on its way to Jamaica, carefully crated and loaded unto the sea vessel carrying it towards its final, permanent abode, high in the misty Blue Mountains.

It was during this time that many apparitions and strange phenomena were taking place throughout the world but mainly in Catholic countries. Portentous signs and wonders mesmerized and befuddled the weeping, worshipful multitudes who would crowd into churches where stone, marble or even wooden statues of the Virgin would be seen to weep copiously at designated hours of the day; or to behold the weird phenomena of the consecrated host in its golden monstrance bleeding a blood-like red fluid before their very eyes.

Many had known of, or even seen for themselves, in emotional visits to Catholic churches in Paris, Lyons and Marseilles, the incorruptible bodies of saintly nuns deceased over many decades, in perfectly preserved state, miraculously exhibiting a truly life-like appearance for all to see.

Then, a few years before, when a construction worker noticed the apparition of the Madonna suspended over the high cusp of Mexico City's main cathedral, he eagerly called the crowd's attention to the beautiful, luminous celestial lady with prayerful hands, seemingly floating precariously above the highest point of the church's structure. He did gesture towards her with his bandaged, almost gangrenous finger which was to be amputated the following day at hospital, due to a crushing work-related injury he had sustained, But then, when he went to hospital the following day for the operation and bandages were removed, the finger was found to be perfectly whole and well.

And so it was, that from Venezuela to far away Japan, and from Yugoslavia to Italy and France, the Virgin Mother made her arresting, phenomenal presence felt. Yet, none of these strange 'miraculous' wonders ever occur in the island of Jamaica. It was left to María Frasca, the Madonna's own selected prophetess, to bring the mystical island and its Bible-loving people under the fold of the Virgin's loving and sorrowful concern.

Mrs. Frasca was continually having visions during which she received clear, auricular and psychic messages from the exquisitely beautiful extra-terrestrial visitor. As she explained in the course of numerous interviews reported in the local and international press, the Madonna would appear unto her with such frequency that she came to regard the visitations as routine occurrences in her life, and she had become accustomed to the welcome state of trance that invariably came upon her every time it happened.

Trance is a sleeplike state, as in deep hypnosis, which appears also in hysteria and in some spiritistic mediums, during which there is limited sensory and motor contact with the ordinary surroundings. It is known that women enter into states of trance with greater ease than men, because women, as a whole, have a lower metabolic rate and a higher parasympathetic output than men. Among many other functions, the parasympathetic nervous system governs reproduction, gestation, and also *the trance states.*

María Frasca did admit that she is very fond of sweets, and it is also known that sweets release tryptophan in the system, an essential amino acid which plays a major role in inducing sleep and trance states, and has been used experimentally in the treatment of insomnia. During trance, an individual's externalized faculties (the five senses) are "detached from the will" allowing the focus of consciousness to be internalized; then, from the intimate connection that exists between the parasympathetic nervous system and trance states, spiritual inspiration emerges... visions and apparitions are seen, voices are heard... all of which are composed of subtle electromagnetic energies not dissimilar to those observed during epileptic seizures. The mind usually returns to its normal condition of equipoise, and the 'visionary experience' then ends.

All of this is fairly well-known among the Catholic priesthood, who are extensively trained in all modalities of psychic phenomena and the spiritual anatomy of man. For this reason, there is a cautious reluctance on the part of the Church's hierarchy to endorse and rush in embrace of seers and visionaries, even when their enthusiastic 'visions' support the Church's dogmas and doctrines.

Then came the climatic event of Mrs. Frasca's visit to Jamaica. A well-publicized press conference at an elegant upscale hotel in the capital city of Kingston, where plans for the erection of the statue of the virgin would be announced, and metaphysical healings would also be conducted by the American psychic, became the occasion for her most dramatic prediction for Jamaica.

For, there she disclosed, that in her most recent vision of the Madonna, the Mother of Jesus had said unto her: "Go and say unto the people of Jamaica, that they are specially beloved by me and that I stand ready to accept the prayers and the pleadings of the suffering, repentant ones, who are prepared to turn away from their sinful ways. And I shall intercede on their behalf with My Son, and He shall have Mercy upon them and turn away the calamities and great disasters that are to come upon the world, for the time of the end is at hand..."

"... and *JAMAICA SHALL BE GREATLY BLESSED, AND LARGE NUMBERS OF PEOPLE FROM MANY LANDS WILL GO TO THAT HOLY ISLAND, FOR THERE IT WILL BE FOUND, IN BLACK FISHES INHABITING JAMAICAN WATERS, THE CURE FOR AN INCURABLE DISEASE...*"

But then, as this Modern Oracle uttered her turbulent and portentous prophetic sayings which she had received in many emotionally and sensually charged visualizations of the Madonna, a vociferous multitude of demonstrators had swiftly gathered at the main entrance of the meeting hall.

The growing throng of placard-bearing Evangelicals, Protestants and members of the Rastafarian faith among others, rubricated their disruption of the Psychic's press conference with the resonant peal of their African drums, punctuated with shouts and chants of... *"WE WANT NO GRAVEN IMAGES IN JAMAICA!" "NO IDOLATROUS WORSHIP OF STATUES IN OUR LAND!" "AWAY WITH IDOLS AND DEMONS!"*

And so, as the tremulous attendants of the foreign visionary's elegant meeting felt their bowels quake and their hearts melt at the sounds of the vehement demonstration outside, the organizers decided to end the press conference and quietly disband, until more favourable circumstances permit an orderly event to take place.

It was later decided not to erect the Virgin's statue at the site in the Blue Mountains, but rather, to discretely install the lifelike marble idol within the safe confines of the Saint Martin of Porres Roman Catholic church in Gordon Town, at the foot of the cool Blue Mountains.

María Frasca returned to the reassuring quietude of her Floridian suburb and did not return to Jamaica, but many here remember her Oracular pronouncements and patiently await their fulfillment. And even though the origin and true source of her visions and celestial messages cannot be firmly ascertained, the fact remains that many of her predictions did prove to be accurate, as in due course they did come to pass. That unspecified "incurable disease" she spoke of in her Jamaican predictive sayings may well be conquered by the tireless efforts of the scientific establishment, or, could well be resurrected from the annals of past secret discoveries. Whichever way it does happen, surely, The Modern Oracle has Spoken... and shall be proven right!

****

Meanwhile, at the Colombian jungle clinic of El Sanatorio, the Cisneros-Valdés medical research team were seeing real evidence of progress, in both, the clinical manifestations as well as in the cytological and antigen-specific laboratory analysis of the test subjects. They were particularly satisfied with the steady improvement shown in the previously desperately ill Maritza Romero Hernández. Her overall clinical picture was nothing short of truly dramatic after almost four months or uninterrupted therapy with the Alchemical ZAM-2RO compound.

And although one of the other patients still remained critically ill due to a sudden unexpected complication arising from an episode of acute post-hemorrhagic anemia, which they were controlling through suitable measures, the general response of the other subjects was most encouraging, especially since every one of them had been terminally ill patients with inoperable tumours of either lung, colon, prostate or the mammary gland. Furthermore, they had at varying stages undergone the standard gamut of anti-cancer therapy available: surgery, radiation, chemotherapy, hormonal therapy, and in a few cases with the then promising Interferon and Monoclonal Antibodies therapy.

Of course, Maritza's case was a particularly challenging one due to the insidious nature and the location of her brain tumour. The gradual but sustained restoration of her psychomotor functions, and the clinical evidence of the shrinking of her distant secondary tumours, demonstrated not only the systemic mode of action and potency of the ZAM-2RO Alchemical compound, but also the fact that it was a benign and effective therapy, for it worked without poisoning the patient, without losing its potency over time, and without killing healthy cells.

In their inter-daily clinical review meetings the research trio made every effort to document all aspects of the trail-blazing medical study they were conducting. The main conclusion they had arrived at was that the ZAM-2RO compound acts as a BRM (Biological Response Modifier), affecting the relationship between the tumour and host, by strengthening the host's biological response to tumour cells. It achieves this through a mechanism of multiple action.

For reasons they could not fully understand, the ZAM-2RO bio-Alchemical compound is highly unstable once it is extracted from its animal source and combined with specific galenicals. It, however, exhibits full, direct antitumour effect when it enters the human subject.

Its multi-pronged attack begins with a severe interference with the tumour cells ability to metastasize and to survive after metastasis, combined with a disruption of the process of neoplastic transformation in cells. In addition to this mode of action at the cellular level, the compound acts in a sustained manner upon immune system imbalances and dysfunctions by modulating, restoring and augmenting the host's normal immunological mechanisms.

Dr. Axel Cisneros Vargas was peculiarly suited to be involved in this dazzlingly sophisticated area of biomedical research, due to his previous extensive work within the realm of *cell mediated immunity.* This normal defense mechanism we have, refers to the immunity conferred by the mutation of the "T Lymphocytes" which occur in the thymus gland. Also known as "T Cells", these lymphocytes directly destroy not only viruses and cells infected with intracellular organisms, but most importantly, they destroy *malignant cells.*

And, as pointed out to me by Dr. Héctor Valdés, they had even received confirmation of these findings from researchers at Mie University in Japan, where they found that in individuals who had suffered a severe deterioration of their immune system, leaving them vulnerable to disease, their thymus gland, which controls the functions of the immune system, had shrunk to half its normal size.

Regardless of the many complexities associated with the ZAM-2RO Alchemical compound's distinctive capabilities for altering biological responses, its fundamental mode of action was to turn patients' immune system against their tumours. It appeared however, to also have the uncanny ability to actually substitute the immune system and act in its place within the subject, in cases where the normal immune mechanism has been damaged and is functioning poorly or not at all.

In the early stages of the secretive clinical trials, the team had to deal with numerous inevitable consequences of previous invasive therapies the patients had received. One of the patients had received radiation to her stomach which created an obstruction in her bowel; she had to undergo abdominal surgery to remove the obstructive mass. Another one of the subjects was still slowly overcoming the ravages of radiation and chemotherapy she had previously received for her advanced breast cancer.

Being almost totally isolated in their far-flung jungle sanctuary, the research team and their assistants had developed a close bond and camaraderie among themselves. Later on, as the condition of the patients gradually improved, that spontaneous fellowship extended its encircling warmth to also embrace them. It was truly the manifestation of the simple childlike friendliness of the peasant folk in the Colombian hinterland.

And those burly 'assistants' who were performing seemingly ordinary tasks around the compound or at the extraction site with the encaged vultures, knew instinctively that they were involved in a very important project... one that had to do with the sick patients in the main building. And, although they were not formally sworn to secrecy, everyone understood the necessity of their being away from their families for extended periods, but also especially, that they were not to discuss with anyone the nature of the work they were engaged in.

Yet, as far away as the large Colombian cities seemed to be from them, they were daily assailed by the arresting realities of the unending internecine slaughter taking place in Medellín, Pereira, Barranquilla or in the sprawling capital city of Bogotá. For, the Colombian authorities had appointed over 2,000 additional secret agents and 24 public prosecutors exclusively dedicated to fight the wave of kidnappings in the country.

And the notorious "Sicarios", those very youthful hit-men operating in the large urban centers, were using garlic-impregnated bullets that are invariably fatal by the septicemia (blood poisoning) produced, once it tears the tissues and comes in contact with the victim's circulating blood. Almost simultaneously, saboteurs working at the behest of leftist guerrilla groups, both, in rural and urban areas, cause electric short-circuits by using a length of wire with weights or stones attached to each end, which is then flung across high tension electric cables, causing major disruptions in the nation's electricity supply.

Dr. Valdés would occasionally join the workers around the bonfire as they sat listening to the news on a radio or just pulsing a guitar to some romantic song. And they would smile knowingly at him, upon hearing the frequently told tale of how Colombian women murder unfaithful husbands in their sleep by means of a smooth nail that is hammered into the top-center area of the skull, with a single, firm impact of the hammer on the nail's head. There is virtually no bleeding-out or any signs of subdural hemorrhage after the nail is pulled out, and the autopsy usually indicates cause of death: Cardiac arrest.

But, Dr. Axel Cisneros would never join them in those moments of casual relaxation. He would be in his minuscule corner of the main administrative area, writing clinical reports or reviewing scientific or medical journals late into the cool mountain nights; and he would be up early in the mornings ready to begin another adventurous day as he carefully monitored the progress and general condition of his precious subjects.

He held very strong opinions regarding the establishment's attitude towards experimental therapies and modes of treatment. In an article he had submitted to one of Colombia's leading newspaper, he stated that, "A government claims that the citizens don't have the right over their bodies when it comes to taking unproven medicines for deadly diseases (like Laetrile for Cancer), yet it gives its citizens the right to poison themselves, and each other, through alcohol, and so forth. The introduction of non-fatal amounts of tobacco by a smoker into another person's body, is no different from lacing someone's food with sub-fatal doses of Arsenic..."

And Axel Cisneros was a true Master of Medical Sciences, often displaying an almost artistic command of his awesome skills. In treating the Acute Posthemorrhagic Anemia occurring suddenly in one of the patients at El Sanatorio, his exquisite and dazzling art became manifest for those present to behold and admire. For, the patient having lost over one third of blood volume in a 24 hour period, was in immediate danger of shock and circulatory collapse.

Dr. Cisneros' first priority was to ensure that his patient's blood pressure did not fall to shock levels. Not having whole blood or plasma immediately available, he opted for the use of large molecular "plasma volume extenders" (dextran) as a temporary blood substitute, while at the same time initiating surgical repair of the arterial erosion which was responsible for the hemorrhagic episode.

It was during those moments of dire emergencies that he would casually go into detailed discourses on some abstruse topic or other, punctuated by brief interruptions as he requested, instructed or directed his assistants in the procedure being carried out. On this occasion he was explaining aspects of the origin of diseases and the classical term, "dyscracia", that was anciently used to signify 'disease'. That old term meant 'an abnormal mixture of the four humours', the same underlying principle of disease processes that was fundamental in Occult Medicine's understanding of the emergence of diseases in living beings.

He patiently explained how all cells have really existed 'from the beginning' and exist today through the mechanism of cell division. But throughout the myriad generations of that cellular division and multiplication, something had happened to adversely affect the smooth genetic mechanism ordained by nature; a kind of 'biological monkey-wrench' had intervened, and the monster cells of Cancer came into being. He also referred to the recent laboratory-induced transformation of normal cells into malignant ones in which 14 mutagenic/mutating steps were identified through which a normal cell becomes a cancerous cell. He felt certain that the same process *in a reverse mode* would likewise transform the cancerous cell into its previous normal state.

And it was well known that no multicelled organism is immune from cancer of one type or another, with the notable exception of the carrion-eating vultures. Even insects get cancer, and many plant forms too, as well as fishes. Contrary to normal cells which have a single small structure at its center, the nucleus; a cancer cell usually exhibits a huge nucleus, and often enough, two or more nuclei. They also show deformed or multiple cell components, and lack the orderly arrangements of normal cells. And of course, the tendency of cancerous cells to proliferate (metastasis) to other parts of the body is perhaps its most salient identifying characteristic and its really menacing feature.

Dr. Héctor Valdés, his sister Josefina, and the team of technicians and assistants closely followed every word uttered by Axel Cisneros, for they were living witnesses to the dramatic, almost unbelievable recovery of each of those erstwhile seriously ill patients who had been given a sure death sentence, as conventional medicine surrendered to the relentless advance of the proliferative cancerous process taking over their bodies.

For, they themselves had seen two of the subjects when they had first arrived at the facility; the chilling words "Cancerous Cachexia" written at the very top of their clinical file indicating the typical chronic wasting, malnutrition and general ill-health seen in advanced Cancer, and from which the common term "wasting disease" originates. Its clinical signs are: inexplicable loss of appetite, slow or dramatic weight loss, toxemia (blood poisoning) and terminal coma.

And so, he would continue his running discourse of medical-scientific knowledge, spanning the centuries from antiquity right unto the most recent discoveries of our times. He then went on to outline how tomato inhibits the growth of prostate cancer by its 'Lycopene', the red pigment carotene of the tomatoes which is also present in other red fruits and berries. It reduces the size of carcinogenic tumours of the prostate and reduce metastasis, the spread of cancer to other tissues of the body, and has a positive effect against cancers of the pancreas, lung and colon.

He had once presented a scientific paper at an international seminar, in which he reported the results of some of his findings on uterine fibroma, popularly known as fibroids. There he reported that these fibrous, encapsulated connective tissue tumours are often caused by excessive proteinization. Benign in nature, they manifest either in a round mass or proliferating seemingly as a vine. Usually, surgery is used, but remissions are very common. It was discovered that over proteinization causes an imbalance in hormonal levels in the affected female, especially of estrogen. He showed how there was an interdependence of protein and sugar in the body's chemistry, so that excessive levels of one creates a physiological craving for the other.

Dr. Cisneros was a firm believer in employing non-blood procedures in medicine and surgery. For, he knew that non-transfusion of blood in cancer patients brings about a better and quicker progress in their restorative process, and they have less recurrence of the disease. The research team itself did not regard the transfusion of blood to be a safe procedure, because blood being a fluid organ of the body and one of its four vital humours, blood transfusion is in reality nothing less than organ transplant, and organ transplant must always be regarded as the last therapeutic option that may be offered to the patient. Furthermore, a high danger of contamination exists when blood donated by individuals who are infected *but have not yet developed antibodies that could be detected* through diagnostic screening tests, is transfused. The risks of disease transmission and immunomodulation are ever present in blood transfusion.

On that occasion, he had ended his veritable *tour de force* with an anecdotal reference to the ancients' use of a type of Kelp or seaweed, 'Laminaria Digitata', which when dried has the ability to rapidly absorb water and expand with considerable force. It was used to dilate the uterine cervical canal in induced abortion, and was so used throughout the centuries in ancient Egypt, Arabia and in parts of Medieval Europe.

In writing his copious notes on the now successful clinical trials with the Alchemical compound ZAM-2RO on advanced cancer patients, he had outlined extensively, the putative mechanism of action of the biological substance. There he explained how the compound effected a realignment of the syncretistic activity of the botanical extracts with the vultures' humoral fluid (gastric). Some of the plant juices act as a catalyst in the cellular binding action of the ZAM-2RO, while others potentiate its carcinolytic, destructive to cancer cells, effects. He had also minutely detailed the carcinophilia or highly destructive affinity of the bio-compound against rapidly multiplying cells.

He had just recently before received an invitation from the prestigious Swedish Academy of Sciences to present his findings at their next plenary meeting, so, he was assiduously organizing his abundant notes and scientific papers on the clinical trials. Yet, in spite of the heady success they were enjoying and the almost celebratory mood that was evident throughout the camp, Dr. Axel Cisneros remained strangely aloof and distant from everyone. To his brother-in-law he had admitted using various hypnagogic/Aphrodisiac herbs such as damiana, ginseng and yohimbe, by which he experienced an intensification of the power of the nervous system and consequent marked emotional pleasure.

He had developed a reckless disregard for what he considered a marred and even warped existence in an imperfect world. And, as Héctor Valdés gradually learnt, his brother-in-law was a deeply troubled man, and apparently had confided in him those intimate matters which he would normally keep to himself. His wife, Josefina, was largely unaware of the causes of his many brooding moments of lonely introspection, and preferring not to interfere, she would quietly await until he eventually pulled himself out of it.

Héctor had become somewhat uneasy when Axel had mentioned that he had doubts as to whether or not it was a useful effort to prolong one's life in a steadily deteriorating "fleshly vehicle" which must be ignominiously shed sooner or later. Both, Héctor and his sister, were not privy to the subjective "life of quiet desperation" that Dr. Cisneros was enduring. His secretive disposition and avuncular manner had always kept everyone, including close family members, unaware of the torments that frequently assailed his mind.

Surely they knew of his chronic depression and the mood of quiescence and stoic fatalism he often indulged in, as on several occasions they found him privately engaged in self-tormenting soliloquies, those enigmatic monologues through which he seemed to be placating the unseen demons inhabiting the dark recesses of his tortured inner world.

And so, it was most of all the odd timing of his sudden and startling action which they had found incomprehensible, beyond any reasonable or logical explanation whatsoever. For, they were at that time savoring the exhilarating, emotional rush of success with the clinical trials they were carrying out.

Axel Cisneros had only said that he was driving out to the nearby township to purchase a few items he needed. One of the workers from El Sanatorio was with him, and they both went into the supply store whose owner was a friend of the Cisneros'. While paying for the supplies and amiably conversing with the proprietor, he noticed a handgun in his friend's waistband, and casually commented that he also intended to purchase one soon.

..."These are the best. Just got it last week; its a .38 calibre revolver... it won't jam or misfire as an automatic pistol would. Here, look at it... its loaded, though," said the proprietor as he carefully handed the firearm to Axel Cisneros who balanced it in his hand, feeling the dull weight of the iron in his palm.

Then, swiftly and unexpectedly, Dr. Cisneros lifted the weapon to his right temple and squeezed the trigger. The deafening explosion coalesced with the shrieking screams of the peasant women in the store, while the other customers stared incredulously at the slumped body of Axel Cisneros, still jerking convulsively like a rag-doll at the hands of a bored child, on the shop's dusty floor.

No one could understand the reasons why he chose to go that way, but more so, the burning question on their lips was, always... *Why at this time?* And in the midst of their acute bereavement and distress, they had to activate the contingency plans that would enable them to continue the bio-alchemical treatment on the subjects, and eventually to wind down the whole operation which was already in its final phases. But, they were then like a rudderless ship on the Ocean which had also lost its captain, and they knew not how they would be able to continue without him...

Chapter 6

Cellular Disrespect for the Limits of Growth

"... a cancer is the uncontrollable multiplication of cells to the mortal detriment of the housing organism..."

*H*ector Valdés wondered what could it be now. He was requested to accompany the prison guard to the office of the Superintendent of the penal institution, and while grooming and getting ready to go, he was reviewing in his mind all the many possibilities that could have prompted this sudden development.

Upon entering the sparcely furnished office, he was cordially welcomed and given a seat. "Valdés, I have good news for you;" said the Superintendent in his customary mellifluous voice.

"We are sending you home... you will be leaving in three days time, on Friday... Do you understand?-*Tres días* only, then, *adiós amigo!* You will be taken from here directly to the airport; be ready for around midday, ok? The flight will be via Panamá; you will be all right. *Comprende Senor?"*

"Yes Sir, comprendo, but why... What happen, Sir?"

"Valdés, the government has decided to release you now, four months before completing your sentence. Your behaviour has been good, you gave us no problems at all. You are a good man, ok? Take good care of yourself now. Goodbye..."

Although he had already acquired a rudimentary understanding of the English language and the gist of what was said to him, the emotional impact of that surprising turn of events in his life, merely added to the confusion and excitement he was experiencing. It was not until the following day that I managed to meet with him, in order to allay his natural fears and unease by explaining to him in detail all aspects of the bureaucratic process that would culminate with his boarding the airplane for Panamá... and freedom, at last. He remained in an unbelieving daze for a long time; then, eventually, when the full force of his impending release from prison dawned in his mind, he realized that he had to quickly formulate plans and set directions for his immediate future out there, in the 'free world'.

Sometime ago, after he had been settled into the daily routine of boredom, dejection and melancholy that marked his extended sojourn at the maximum security facility, I had managed to persuade him of the wisdom of returning to his family in Bolivia rather than to start all over again in Colombia. Eventually, after much thought, he gradually reestablished communication with his wife, his daughters and with Julio, his son. They were all anxiously awaiting his return, and even reassured him that no one over there knew anything about 'the problem', for they were all told that he was in the United States and would soon be returning home.

He wanted to make a complete break with his past, and often dreamt of regaining his prestige and good name in his hometown of Santa Cruz, where he would again reactivate the biomedical laboratory he had left behind and generally, return to the placid, somnolent life he enjoyed amidst his own people, before he had ventured into the hostile outside world of runaway ambitions, fast money and illicit drugs.

When I enquired about his plans for continuing research into the Alchemical cure for Cancer, the ZAM-2RO compound, and all the accumulated clinical data on the trials he participated in, his enigmatic response was..." I am too old and tired for all that now. Why don't you pursue it? You have all the necessary information to do it, and I am leaving the entire file with you... I really don't want to take it along with me. I need to forget the past and get along with my life... my family also needs me..."

He reminded me once more, that I should try by all means, to contact the Cuban Doctor who had worked for sometime with his brother-in-law Axel in southern Africa, and who had also done considerable experimental work with the bio-alchemical anticancer compound. He urged me to make all efforts to get in touch with this medical researcher from Cuba who could not only corroborate the efficacy and safety of the compound, but would also definitely be able to assist with any efforts to replicate the successful Cisneros-Valdés clinical trials.

I accepted all the information offered, along with the voluminous files, photographs, medical and laboratory records, and a variety of notes and other material, wondering all the time if it would ever be of any practical use, or even, if I would ever do anything about it... because it all seemed then so far-fetched and improbable; or so I thought at that time.

We did keep in touch for sometime after Héctor had left Jamaica, and he seemed to be getting along pretty well back home. Gradually, our correspondence became infrequent and far apart, until at length we lost track of each other. The last I did hear from him, however, was that the family was planning to relocate in the city of Cochabamba and might do so soon afterwards.

****

Many years had passed by with its increasingly compact flow of events in our lives, and the memory of Héctor Valdés became part of a dim past that has been crowded out by the daily drag of modern living with all its cares and preoccupations substituting our former lofty, idealistic objectives.

Then, sometime near the end of 1996, I was asked to organize and coordinate the visit to Jamaica of Their Imperial Highnesses, Ethiopian Princes Ermias Sahle Selassie and Bekere Fikre Selassie, the grandsons of Ethiopian Emperor Haile Selassie. That week-long, heavily-scheduled series of events, official visits, receptions and press conferences turned out to be fortuitously important in terms of the reactivation of the Alchemical Cure for Cancer.

That unforgettable and intensely hectic tour began with the arrival from New York of the Royal visitors and their security detail at the Jamaican capital's international airport. Crowds of adoring, worshipful members of the Rastafarian faith had from earlier on jampacked the terminal's main building, and were intent, amidst the heavy security, to get a glimpse or even a slight touch of these descendants of the former Ethiopian monarch whom they revere as the 'Living God'.

With some difficulty we managed to get them through the multitude and into the waiting vehicles which then sped away to the uptown Pegasus Hotel, where an entire upper floor had been designated for the illustrious visitors and their entourage. The motorcade had, however, grown to some thirty-five or more vehicles, as a good part of the airport crowd had decided to follow us to wherever we were going.

Things had been organised thoroughly, so that upon arrival at the hotel we all went straight to the top floor, leaving the swelling crowd downstairs in the main lobby. The floor had been sealed off and the elevators were manned by security personnel from the government's intelligence arm, the Special Branch. Soon enough though we had a number of people milling around in the corridors and coming to the suite's main entrance seeking audience with Their Highnesses.

Just as I was making alternate security arrangements to ensure an orderly flow of visitors and well-wishers, I was approached by two white-clad members of the 'Twelve Tribes of Israel', one of several Mansions or organisations that make up the many groupings within the Nation of Rastafari in Jamaica.

"We came to see Prince Ermias, Sir,... at his request." said one of them, while giving me a pleasant smile.

"Kindly identify yourself". I quietly replied.

Then, with a beaming smile and a twinkle in his eyes, he replied; "I see that you don't remember me, eh? I am Dr. Carlton Fraser. It has been such a long time... Have I changed that much?'

Instantly recognizing that friend of old, we both embraced and exchanged pleasantries and a few memories from way back then.

"I have been assigned as personal physician to Their Highnesses during their stay in Jamaica. But, this is really an unexpected coincidence... Where have you been all this time...?"

And it had really been a very long time since we last saw each other; over twelve years. Dr. Fraser was no longer working within the government services, but was now in private practice and also acting as Medical Consultant to the Ethiopian Royal family now living in exile in Europe and North America; and so, he travelled frequently and extensively.

Then, amidst many constant interruptions, schedule reviews, appointment confirmations and calls from various entities, we managed to hold some semblance of communication going between us. For, the entire organizing team of some twenty or so persons was labouring under constant and demanding circumstances, having to deal with myriad unpredictable and unruly groups and individuals who are burdened with gigantic egos and an insatiable desire to be in the limelight of prominence and attention. Then surely, the inevitable gamut of intrigues, misinformation and downright sabotage that seem to follow the Royal entourage with its trail of groupies and assorted sycophants, just made our task that much more challenging and difficult.

The wide ranging and intense tour schedule for the Royal visitors saw the motorcade travelling wide and far throughout the island, but we ensured that there would be the obligatory rest periods and a whole day free of any official activities or appearances. And it was during those few leisure moments in an otherwise hectic timetable of activities, that Dr. Fraser and I remembered our mutual friend Dr. Héctor Velarde Valdés and the rare knowledge he freely shared with us. In the meantime, their Highnesses had accepted a luncheon invitation for this 'free day', and so, in a reduced caravan of some six cars, we easily motored on towards *Mount Zion*. The beautiful, green rolling hills and smooth flatlands of *Mount Zion*, the thousandacre coconut plantation owned by the colourful personage Prince Charles Brown, was the impressive setting for the rural luncheon in honour of the Ethiopian visitors. Its centerpiece was the historic Great House, formerly the residence of slavemasters during the dark period of British chattel slavery in Jamaica. For, the estate was in those historic days one of the largest holdings in the parish of Saint Ann, and still had relics of its brutal past, like the minidungeons for punishing slaves, whipping posts and sundry chains and manacles scattered about the place.

And as Dr. Fraser and I reminisced on various aspects of the Alchemical treatment for Cancer, he frankly voiced his opinion about the possibilities of success with an attempted replication of the South American clinical experience. He emphasized the urgency of carrying out any evaluation of a potential cure for Cancer, no matter how unorthodox it may be, for, recent statistics released by the World Health Organization reveal that by the year 2,020 it is estimated that some *10 million persons per year* will be affected by various types of Cancer.

But then, Dr. Fraser had a profound understanding of the mechanism of action of the bio-Alchemical compound, for, he had worked with several experimental cancer treatments whose principal mode of action was by immunomudulation, that is, direct activity upon the efficiency of the body's immune system. He also strongly believed that the bio-Alchemical treatment would likewise be effective against the HIV-AIDS syndrome because of its mode of action.

And we continued throughout the numerous activities associated with the often tumultuous visit of the Ethiopian Princes, exchanging ideas and impressions on all aspects of the Alchemist's abstruse science, until we finally agreed to hold a formal meeting to definitely formulate strategies and a plan of action to replicate the Cisneros-Valdés clinical study. Everything would be done right here in Jamaica, under cover of strict secrecy.

And so, we went about quietly laying down plans to conduct the clinical trials at that remote rural site nestled between the imposing mountain ridges of Northwest Jamaica. We decided to try to enlist the assistance of international research centers involved in the fight against Cancer, and to explore the possibility of obtaining technical and financial aid from private sources and foundations sympathetic to our objectives.

Subsequent meetings saw a gradual crystallization of the procedural aspects of the project, for which a manual of procedures and techniques would be prepared. There was a tangible, almost palpable excitement permeating those quiet working sessions at the Great House, with each participant freely contributing to the shaping of the planned project.

Dr. Fraser had on this occasion shared with us some of his experiences with his most celebrated patient, the world-renowned reggae prophet and visionary Bob Marley. The Cancer that was taking its toll on the popular poet-singer had metastasized to distant parts of his body including the brain. They had taken him to the prestigious Sloan Kettering Memorial Centre in New York, where gallant efforts were being made to save Marley's life, but he kept on steadily deteriorating, becoming weaker and emaciated.

Carlton Fraser described how he could actually 'see' the ebbing life-force steadily slipping away from his friend and patient, and felt truly helpless and inadequate at not being able to do more to save him. And, while restlessly pacing the floor in the room where Bob had been placed, he noticed a sheet of paper almost beneath the bed. He casually picked it up and saw that it was a promotional flyer announcing a lecture for that very evening by the renowned German cancer specialist Dr. Josef Issels.

He immediately decided that he would attend, and once there, made every effort to speak with Dr. Issels, who agreed to treat Bob Marley at his private clinic in Germany. The malignancy that had taken hold of his patient had already invaded vital organs and continued to shed off malignant cells which would migrate to distant parts of the body, establishing new, fatal colonies of neoplasmic monster cells growing without restraint. This was the seeming ineluctable process of Cancer that had forced him to constantly breathe in the suffocating air of death, the central rottenness of which was the ugly mass of grapebunch-like tissue that was the large tumour masses in lung and brain that had clamped its vice-grip upon his friend.

In spite of the valiant efforts of Dr. Issels and his team in Germany, Bob's deterioration continued its downward trend, until sometime after, defeat was acknowledged, and he was sent back home... to die. He didn't make it to Jamaica though, dying instead in Miami, another victim of "the crablike pestilence which no man cureth..."

And Dr. Fraser frequently ruminated over that dramatic episode in his professional life, for he was a close friend and confidant of Bob Marley. In casual conversations at the Great House he continued to ponder on the vagaries of cruel fate, for, as he did say to us then, had he known of the Alchemical bio-compound in those days he would have certainly tried it. "Without official sanction? Would you have done it in secret?" I asked of him. "I would have done *anything* to save him!"

He then reaffirmed his willingness to replicate the Cisneros-Valdés clinical trials right here in Jamaica, and for which he has at least four candidates, advanced Cancer patients who would be most willing to undergo any experimental treatment that offers the slightest hope for their desperate condition.

A few weeks later, during one of our technical planning meetings, we did a comprehensive review of current Cancer diagnostic and therapeutic procedures and the level of success attained with them. And at these stimulating brain-storming sessions we learnt among many other things, that the mimetic character of potentially cancerous cells seem to mask the actuating factor that causes normal cells to be 'startled' into unprecedented activity, and as Cancer is really a DNA (a complex protein, carrier of genetic information) disease, that is, an abnormality of the genes occurring at the molecular level, its cure would likely involve a substance which acts upon the genetic material to restore the DNA molecule to its former state of "normality'.

It is also known that very low concentrations of DNA are chemically amplified by a simple procedure of repeatedly heating and cooling the DNA. With each of these *hot and cold cycles,* the number of molecules present is doubled. Infinite generations of exact copies of the original DNA are thus created.

An alteration of the cyclic pattern of regular heat and cold changes, would bring about a severe irregularity in the genetic material, setting the normal cell on its way to becoming a cancerous cell. As outlined in the Cisneros-Valdés clinical reports, one of the modes of action of the bio-alchemical compound is to restore the regular *hot and cold cycle* at the cellular level, thereby reversing the mutation process of DNA and bringing about normality.

The recent dramatic increase in the incidence of Cancer has been traced to the current high levels of environmental chemical toxicity that comes with the 'advances' of modern life through Science and Technology.

The multiplicity of synthetic chemicals around us, are an important factor in the chain of carcinogenic substances which we absorb into our bodies. An example of this is the fuel additive MTBE (Methyl tertiary Butyl ester), a powerful, complex chemical, that enhances combustion in car engines and cuts toxic vehicle emissions. Yet, that selfsame additive is known to be a potential carcinogen which has leaked from tens of thousands of underground gasoline storage tanks and contaminated aquifers and various groundwater sources.

Furthermore, even the most careful screen-testing of chemicals and drugs cannot always reveal the possibility that a drug might produce either immediate or long term unexpected harmful effects, because laboratories cannot, for example, fully simulate a chemical's behaviour in the diverse and complex outside world. This world outside the laboratory is already saturated with thousands of different synthetic chemicals, many of which can, and do, interact with each other as well as with living things.

And, although some of these substances are innocuous on their own, if they join together, whether inside or outside our bodies, can produce new, toxic compounds. What makes this threat so exquisitely insidious and deceptive, is the fact that certain of these chemicals become toxic, and even carcinogenic, *only after the body's metabolism processes them.*

Then, as mundane sciences have almost exhausted the Nazi-German body of various physiologic, toxic and chemical experimental data obtained from concentration camp human "guinea-pigs", reliance is now placed almost entirely, on the standard method of administering a measured dose of drug or chemical to laboratory animals, and then try to apply by means of extrapolation, the results to human beings.

This methodology though, is inherently unreliable because different animals often react quite differently to various chemicals and toxins. For example, it is known that a small dose of the highly toxic "Dioxin" will readily kill a female guinea pig by percutaneous absorption, but that same dose has to be increased 5,000 times to kill a hamster. Even closely related species like rats and mice react differently to many chemicals. It is obvious then, that researchers cannot be certain that a particular drug or chemical will be safely tolerated by humans.

Even those laboratories now experimenting with testing chemicals on cultured human cells, will have no sure predictor of the reactions or long-term deleterious effects of toxins, drugs and chemicals on human beings, since they would not be getting an environmentally 'true' picture, 'in vivo', of the tested substance interacting in a 'real life' environment.

And, as the team continued their panoramic review and evaluation of the many known and hypothetical causes of Cancer, attention was drawn to the fact that many of these 'precursor' or 'trigger' carcinogenic substances that are barely detected in water, become concentrated in astounding amounts in the final recipients down the line in the food-chain continuum, such as: fishes, mollusca, farm and domestic animals, and even fruits and vegetables to a lesser extent, to finally rest within the human organism with their terrible sequelae of pathogenic effects.

The very insidious toxic effects of certain chemicals have only recently been uncovered and reported in the specialized journals. We now know, for example, that PCB's (Polychlorinated biphenyls) which have been in widespread use since the early 1930's, consisting of over two hundred aliphatic (oily) compounds used in pesticides, plastics, lubricants, detergents, electrical insulation and other products, along with dioxins and DDT residues among others, are now classified as *endocrine disrupters.*

When taken into the body, these *endocrine disrupters* masquerade as natural hormones, interfering with their regulating functions, by either imitating them in harmful ways or blocking them. They also have the potential to actually disrupt the normal functions of the body's entire endocrine system, the source of hormones.

The uncanny ability of some of these chemicals to readily mimick the female sex hormone estrogen, has recently been blamed for the increased prevalence of precocious puberty among young girls. This in turn, has been linked to consumption of meat from animals raised on a variety of growth stimulating compounds. Still, others were claiming that estrogen-containing hair products, as well as many other environmental chemicals that also mimic estrogen, were the offending agents.

It had been known for sometime now, that chemical toxins severely weaken immune systems, rendering individuals highly susceptible to viral infections, but, most critically, there were indications that many of these 'hormone mimicking' chemical toxins are the direct cause of the relatively recent dramatic increase in the incidence of *hormonally sensitive* or *hormonally mediated* cancers in both men and women. The now ubiquitous breast, testicular and prostate cancers show an obvious affinity for these adipose (fatty) glandular organs which are hormonally regulated, and are therefore, more amenable to the devastating carcinogenic action of the 'endocrine disrupters'.

And so we continued through many months, that core working team of four, eagerly outlining plans, formulating procedures and resolving multiple logistics and practical issues related to the proposed clinical study we were about to embark on. We soon realized, however, that we would have to go it alone, for, the international cancer research fraternity totally ignored our proposals for joint collaborative efforts in testing and evaluating the anti-cancer effects of the bio-alchemical compound. This of course, did not discourage us at all, and we held fast to our original resolve to carry out the clinical trials regardless of the obstacles and setbacks we may encounter.

****

Another year slipped by with all the intensity of a belly-churning roller-coaster ride, the rapidity and frequency of everyday events with its copious changes giving many of us the impression that 'time is moving so fast'...

I was then barely enjoying a kind of 'working Sabbatical', which meant pounding away at an old electronic typewriter, trying to meet one or another seemingly capricious deadline set by my publisher. Safely ensconced in a remote corner of southern Jamaica amidst the thick verdant foliage of nature and the crystalline azure of the nearby sea, I was surely insulated from the constant, nagging cares of the maddening city lifestyle.

The ZAM-2RO clinical study was still in a dormant state, not having yet gotten off the ground; I began wondering if the complexities and challenges we were facing had dampened the fires of enthusiasm that were so evident in all participants at the inception. Our contacts had become sporadic and far between; and the constant absence from Jamaica due to international travel demands of Dr. Fraser, further contributed to the general feeling of dormancy we were all experiencing in respect of the project.

But, after being there for only three months or so, I allowed a good friend and former colleague to persuade me to take a teaching position at a large rural area High School. His rationale for the request was that they "desperately needed" a Tutor in languages for their senior groups, and of course, he thought only of me. He further assured me that I would have time available for my writing since I would be on the morning shift, with afternoons free. He, being the Principal for the institution, would see to it that everything would be just fine for me.

I was really trading one deep rural region of Jamaica, near to its encircling sea, for another still deeper rural setting, but this time it was a truly mountainous backwater in the remote hinterland parish of Trelawny, a region rich in the slavery-days plantation history of Jamaica and its heroic, unconquered Maroon freedom fighters.

Travelling through its winding and narrow mountain roads, I quietly enjoyed the effortless, majestic beauty of green-carpeted hillsides and brilliant lapis lazuli skies. And I continued thereafter to always marvel at the spectacular view of far reaching misty hills, all bristling with the ubiquitous vertical 'Yam-sticks', upon which the climbing vine wraps itself, as it avidly seeks the photosynthetic alchemy of sunlight to stimulate its nourishing life-sustaining sap.

Upon arrival at the Albert Town High School I was surprised to find that my friend, the Principal, was no longer there, but had gone on pre-retirement leave; he certainly did not tell me about his imminent departure! Nevertheless, I was kindly attended to by the acting vice-principal who promptly informed me that I would definitely need a Medical Certificate of Health before I could take up duties. A bit dismayed, I asked if that would necessitate me going back to the nearest township to seek a doctor for the certificate. "Oh no Sir, you can just go down to Ulster Spring, some five miles from here, to Dr. Davis the District Medical Officer. He will give you a certificate. He takes care of all our teachers;" replied the helpful school official, who later on also made arrangements for me to be settled into the spartan living quarters I had been assigned to.

Albert Town is a quaint, sleepy agricultural village at the edge of the famous 'Cockpit Country', the primeval, rocky mountainous reserve of untouched beauty, where its sheer stone cliffs and numerous miles-long caves became the historic scenario of the Maroons ignominious defeat of the British colonial forces in the eighteenth century. A quiet town of gentle folk, I was bemused to note that there wasn't even a Police station there, the nearest one being at Ulster Spring.

I motored down to the town of Ulster Spring and entered a true time-warp; it was like going back to the 1940's, as everything there was ancient and decrepit; really out of touch with the times. The local 'hospital' consisted of two small wood and stone buildings badly in need of a coat of paint. The whole place was so quiet and deserted. I walked through the silent corridors and eventually found a ward attendant who told me that Dr. Davis would soon be in office.

True enough, I was shortly after greeted by a jovial old gentleman whose manner was friendly and inviting. We chatted informally for a while, then he casually wrote up the certificate for me. "Oh, you are Spanish, eh? One of your countrymen works here too. He's not in today, he's doing duty at the clinic in Jackson Town, but he'll be here tomorrow. I'd like you to meet him, he's a very nice fellow."

"I would be delighted to meet him, for sure. Where is he from?" I asked.

"Dr. Amable is from Cuba. He's been here with us for the past three years more of less..." Dr. Davis replied.

Surprised, I instantly flashed back... "What did you say his name was?" "We all call him 'Amable' which is his first name; none of us can pronounce his surname, he replied, laughing out aloud."

"I will return tomorrow, Dr. Davis. I certainly would like to meet Dr. Amable; it's quite a while since I last spoke Spanish;" I said, while thinking about this uncanny coincidence, for, I distinctly remembered that the name of the Cuban researcher who had worked alongside Dr. Axel Cisneros in Africa, was also 'Amable' which in the Spanish language means "kind".

It wasn't until some ten days later that I managed to pay a return visit to the museum-like hospital in Ulster Spring, and had to wait for a few minutes until Dr. Davis came for me and took me to meet Dr. Amable. And there he was, in a dingy little corner office, seated at a wooden table; a rustic examination bed was the only other furniture in the sparsely furnished 'consulting room'.

He rose and gave me a warm welcome, repeatedly stating how happy he was to meet a Spanish speaking person in this remote area of Jamaica. I could see that he was truly elated with my visit, and so, we conversed casually on a number of topics, intermingled with snippets of information about ourselves and the work we were each engaged in. An easy and sincere friendship quickly developed between us, and in subsequent visits Dr. Amable freely spoke about himself, his family and the extensive professional experience he had acquired over many years of medical service in numerous countries.

Gradually, I had come to the realization that he was indeed the Dr. Amable that Héctor Valdés had told me about, but it was not until some time after we had met that I decided to bring up the subject matter of the bio-alchemical Cancer treatment and the projected clinical trials on it in which I was involved. My extreme caution was due to my keen understanding of the stifling and paranoid atmosphere of suspicion and mistrust that characterises the totalitarian society he came from.

But Amable was far above that level of human misery and indignity, and often reminded me that he was a 'free thinker'. He had spent over sixteen years in Angola, Mozambique, Senegal and Zambia as a Medical team leader, and had become a Professor of the Swahili language, and an expert in Occult Medicine and African Healing Systems.

He was Dr. Amable Thaureaux-Bataille, M.D.; a graduate of the University of Havana and specialist in Internal Medicine. And yes, he was quite knowledgeable in the fields of Traditional, Occultic and Alchemical Medicine. He instantly remembered Dr.

Axel Cisneros whom he had met in Zimbabwe, and was really surprised when I told him about his tragic death in Colombia.

As we continued to grow in friendship and mutual respect for each other, he spontaneously shared with me the rich and varied experiences he had accumulated over his long professional trajectory. Here in Jamaica he had seen many of the tropical diseases he encountered during his long medical sojourn in southern Africa. Of course, he didn't expect to find cases of Priapism, the abnormal, painful and continued erection of the penis caused by Leishmaniasis or cancerous elephantiasis, because the local folk here frequently indulge their penchant for 'washouts' with strong cathartic purgatives, which obviates the onset of many parasitic infestations.

He confirmed the dramatic cures of various forms of cancer which he himself had witnessed in Africa, with the use of traditional Occult methods where animal and plant extracts are combined in secret decoctions whose actions are systemic and complete. He attested to numerous cures with these bio-compounds in cases of acute lymphatic leukemia, various carcinomas, brain tumours, lung, prostatic and colo-rectal cancers.

During the lengthy period he was in Africa, he had worked alongside many great physicians who routinely combined their western training with traditional and Occult methods in a variety of critical and life-threatening situations. He himself had used Professor Charles Ssali's botanical extract "Mariandina" in many cases of Cancer and *HIV/AIDS* with virtually 100% success. Ssali is a Ugandan physician with decades-long experience in the preparation and use of botanical bio-extracts to treat advanced systemic Cancer.

A few months later, in one of our many lively discussions on the intricacies and abstruse character of many of these 'exotic' therapies, we were joined by Dr. Davis, the SMO (Senior Medical Officer) at the hospital, who although trained in the traditional Western school of medicine at Howard University, was nevertheless quiet conversant with the Arcana of Occult Medicine and Alchemy.

On this occasion we were casually talking in Dr. Davis' surgery, when Amable in his quaintly accented English explained the mechanism of action of the bio-alchemical compound. "Its systemic action brings about a gradual reduction of metastasized cells and colonies throughout the body with a concomitant increase in the activity and efficiency of the immune system. It actually restores the immune system. Seeing it work, is a true manifestation of the process of 'epiphylaxis', the induced increase in the defensive powers of the body..." I found his succinct words eerily reminiscent of those of Dr. Héctor Valdés many years before, when he was outlining to me the strange mode of action of the ZAM-2RO compound.

I recalled then, some comments made to me by Dr. Fraser when I first mentioned the bio-alchemical compound and the Colombian clinical experience. "I have stayed clear of these Occult cures of the Alchemists, because of a disturbing episode we lived through with one of my patients some years ago right here in Jamaica..."

"Some experimental anti-cancer medication was sent to me from Italy, and I decided to put it to the test. It worked marvelously and soon enough the patient I had on it was virtually free from Cancer; but then, after a while I just couldn't get any more of the medication. The doctor who had sent it to me had no more, and couldn't get any more either..., he himself had gotten it from another supplier elsewhere, and so it went on".

"And then the Cancer came back, fulminating like a wildfire. We tried everything possible but the patient died some eight weeks later... there was nothing further that we could have done for him."

When I related this incident to them, Dr. Amable smiled enigmatically and said, "That is precisely where the fatal mistake is made. Its action is systemic and gradual, it works over a period of time and therefore necessitates considerable patience on the part of the clinician. The treatment must be administered continuously for at least 6 to 18 months. See, it really isn't a 'medicine' in the traditional sense of the word. Here we are really dealing with 'living substances', or biological fluids that were known to

172

the Alchemists of old as the 'bodily humours' whose mechanism of action is entirely different to that of the inert substances we know as medicines."

And he went on to outline the *carcinolytic* action of the compound whereby it is destructive to cancer cells, and the *carcinophilic* behaviour that it exhibits, that is, its marked affinity for malignant and rapidly multiplying cells.

Dr. Amable Thaureaux-Bataille was married to a Jamaican citizen and they had four grown children, one of whom was also a physician in Cuba. And although his wife had been living in Cuba for over thirty years, she had not adopted that country's nationality, neither had she given up her Jamaican one. His official salary as a physician in Cuba was 400 Cuban pesos equivalent to US$20, which his family receives monthly on his behalf.

In order to get the privilege of being posted overseas he 'volunteered' to donate half of his working hours free, so he officially earns half of a physician's salary in the government service in Jamaica. But, as every Cuban worker posted overseas is obligated to do, he must religiously turn over half of his salary to the Cuban embassy in Kingston, so that he was really working in Jamaica as a full-time Resident and Consultant within the government services at *one quarter* the regular salary of his Jamaican colleagues. And although Dr. Amable was constantly being asked by prominent physicians in the area to join them in their lucrative private practice on a part-time basis, he always declined, for he would have to turn over half of those earnings to his government.

He had long ago become disenchanted and embittered over the corruption and heartlessness of the communist system in his country. He told us of an incident there of which he himself had firsthand knowledge. A desperately ill child with a relatively rare form of stem cell leukemia, needed a medication which was available in the USA. Distant relatives in Florida arranged for it to be sent through a friend, then called to advise them to collect it. But, unfortunately, and tragically, that telephone call was intercepted by operatives of Cuba's dreaded secret police, the G-

2, who immediately sent someone to the designated address and collected the medication long before the rightful person came for it. Of course, the cruel interceptors would sell the medicine on the black market with no thought or remorse for the young life they had imperilled.

I had often thought about the strange turns of fate which had caused me to accept that teaching position in Albert Town, placing me in the unique situation where I actually met and consulted extensively with this knowledgeable and sensitive professional who had considerable experience with the Alchemical bio-extract in the treatment of Cancer.

We did not see each other for some two months after that, due to our varied conflicting obligations at work and home. Then, at the end of the yearly Christmas holidays, I went to Ulster Spring to visit once more with my friendly Latin compatriot. He told me then that he was supplementing his meagre income by doing obstetrics sessions at the maternity wards of two nearby parish hospitals; and he was in high spirits and looked so much better than he did previously.

It was only then that I related to him our plans to replicate the Cisneros-Valdés clinical trials here in Jamaica, and the advanced state of readiness we had so far achieved. He listened attentively and with great interest as I carefully detailed the overall objectives of the trials, its procedural stages and the techniques to be employed. I went on to formally invite him to join the research team in carrying out the projected study, and to participate with us on an equal footing in all aspects of the enterprise.

After a long pause, during which Dr. Amable seemed to be weighing my proposal in his mind, he replied by saying, "I certainly would be delighted to be a part of the research team, but really, I must decline your offer, for, the whole thing could be legally, ethically or morally reprehensible to carry out." "What do you mean by that, in what way would it be objectionable?" I asked.

He looked me straight in the eye, and asked, "Will the patient or their families be informed as to exactly what the medications they will be getting consists of... I mean, the substances... how they are obtained and from what sources they come from?"

"No, of course not. It is not necessary for them to know all that. The protocol in our Manual of Procedures pointedly forbids disclosing that, but furthermore they are not interested in such technicalities; they only want to know that a cure will be achieved," I replied in turn.

Dr. Amable smiled pleasantly while responding, "Sounds really interesting... fascinating I should say. I will let you know soon what is decided about that, ok?... When will the team begin its work?"

Epilogue

$\mathcal{W}$e had written to a number of Cancer research institutes in several countries seeking to establish a collaborative joint effort in confirming the efficacy and safety of the bio-alchemical anti tumour compound. This was deemed necessary before embarking on clinical trials involving human subjects.

Although many of the prospective cancer patients who had been pre-selected to participate in the trials have already died, we nevertheless decided to have the compound tested 'in vitro' for its effect on the ectopic expression and proliferation of tumour cells before attempting to use it 'in vivo'.

The single positive response to our proposal came from the prestigious Max Planck Institute for Experimental Medicine, in Germany. They offered to test our bio-compound (BRM, Biological Response Modifier) on their ion-channel in a cell-culture system. Mammalian cancer cells for the experimental cell-culture would be obtained by cloning and expressing them from rat brain, mouse brain and from bovine retina.

Another phase of the tests would involve human cell lines taken from breast carcinoma, breast invasive ductal carcinoma, melanoma cells and prostate cancer cells. The main cellular event to be measured is the proliferation of cancer cell lines in the solution (Oncogenic potential of cell cycle-regulated $K+$ channel) after coming in contact with our BRM. In fact, the results of these tests in Germany would determine the future of the clinical trails we hope to conduct here in Jamaica.

We are, however, often besieged by a sense of 'stalled urgency' regarding the projected clinical trials. Its as if time has accelerated its inexorable future march with so many cancer victims in our midst who continue to die in excruciating agony and pain. Nevertheless, each stage in the testing and development of the Alchemical Cure for Cancer must, by necessity, be carried out systematically and thoroughly, in order to obviate the numerous pitfalls that were encountered by many of those intrepid pioneers who preceeded us.

This continuing saga and exciting adventure in the quest for the 'natural' Cancer cure will go on in spite of the many obstacles facing us. The narrative of our relentless search and preparation for the projected clinical trials will be chronicled in detail in the upcoming sequel to this volume, and will be entitled *"Cancer Alchemy in Jamaica."*

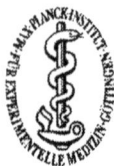

MAX-PLANCK-INSTITUT
FÜR EXPERIMENTELLE MEDIZIN
Abteilung Molekulare Biologie Neuronaler Signale

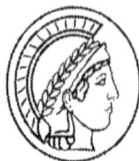

MPI für exp. Medizin, Hermann-Rein-Str. 3, D-37075 Göttingen

Dr. Miguel F. Brooks
Radiance
5 Main Street
POB 421
Mandeville
Jamaica, W.I.

Direktor:
Prof. Dr. Walter Stühmer

Hermann-Rein-Str. 3
D-37075 Göttingen

Telefon: +49-551-3899-646/648
Telefax: +49-551-3899-644
E-mail: wsluehm@gwdg.de

November 29, 2000
ws-ri

Dear Dr. Brooks,

Thank you for your kind letter dated 6th of Nov. 2000, and please excuse my belated reply. I read with great interest about your work. Unfortunately, we are not in a position of directly helping you. However, let me suggest something different. We are also working on possible treatments against cancer based on a novel function for an ion channel that we have described for the first time (see attachments). This seems to be general principle, but the mechanism is unknown. There is a (albeit speculative) possibility that your BRM´s interact with our ion channel. If this would be the case, we would want to collaborate with you, since this would be of mutual interest. At this point let me state clearly that this would be a true collaboration, and that the BRM´s would (and by all means) remain your (Jamaica's) property. I am stating this because I strongly oppose the stealing of natural compounds and traditional products from other countries, and I consider my above statement as obvious.

How shall we proceed? We are not clinically oriented, and therefore cannot make any clinical trials. We would test your BRMs on our ion channel in a cell-culture system. We would test for action on the ion channel and its effect on cell proliferation of cancer cell lines in culture. I guess this would be the first step and the future would depend on the outcome of these experiments. We would of course cover all the costs involved. What is your opinion?

Sincerely yours,

i. a. H. Rennert

Walter Stühmer

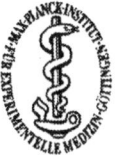

MAX-PLANCK-INSTITUT
FÜR EXPERIMENTELLE MEDIZIN

Abteilung Molekulare Biologie Neuronaler Signale

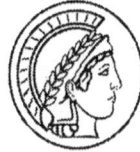

MPI für exp. Medizin, Hermann-Rein-Str. 3, D-37075 Göttingen

Dr. Miguel F. Brooks
Radiance
5 Main Street
POB 421
Mandeville
Jamaica, W.I.

Direktor:
Prof. Dr. Walter Stühmer

Hermann-Rein-Str. 3
D-37075 Göttingen

Telefon: +49-551-3899-646/648
Telefax: +49-551-3899-644
E-mail: wstuehm@gwdg.de

March 13th, 2001
ws-ri

Dear Dr. Brooks,

thank you for your reply of December 29th, and please excuse for my belated answer.

For the patch-clamp measurements we would require only a minimal quantity of the substance you would like us to test. The system we use is to record from a single cell in a volume of about 0.5 ml. Therefore we would only need enough substance to obtain an effective dose in volume of a few milliliters. I assume that you would be able to provide us with this sample in a few months. We are assuming it is water-soluble. When ready, you can send it to us via parcel service (courier) and we will pay the freight costs involved.

With my best regards,

Walter Stühmer

179

Bibliography

Further reading on topics covered in this work may be found in the following partial listing of sources and references, some of which are however, rare, out-of-print books.

J. L. Henderson & M. Oakes, *The Wisdom of the Serpent*, George Braziller, Inc. 1951

Enrique Cornelio Agrippa, *Filosofía Oculta*, Editorial Kier, Buenos Aires, Argentina 1929

Félix Martí-Ibanez, *Essays on the History of Medical Ideas*, MD Publications, New York, 1979

Franz Hartmann, *The Life of Paracelsus*, Routledge & Kegan Paul, Ltd. 1936

E. A. W. Budge, *The Divine Origin of the Craft of the Herbalist*, London, 1928

G. L. Williams, *Priestess of the Occult, Madame Blavatsky*; Alfred Knopf, New York, 1946

Alvin Kuhn, *Theosophy, A Modern Revival of Ancient Wisdom*; H. Holt & Co., New York 1930

James H. Breasted, *Ancient Records of Egypt*, London, 1907

Walter A. Jayne, *Healing Gods of Ancient Civilization*, New Haven, CT 1925

Eliphas Levi, *El Gran Arcano del Ocultismo Revelado*, Editorial Kier, Buenos Aires, Argentina, 1963

Eliphas Levi, *El Libro de los Esplendores*, Editorial Kier, Buenos Aires, Argentina. 1970

Dr. Isador Kalish (Translator) *Sepher Yezirah, A Book on Creation or the Jewish Metaphysics of Remote Antiquity*; Rosicrucian Press, 1966

Aldo Lavagnini, *El Secreto Masónico*; Editorial Kier, Buenos Aires, Argentina. 1963

Rodman R. Clayson, *Egypt's Ancient Heritage*, Supreme Grand Lodge of AMORC, Calif. 1971

AMORC, *Rosicrucian Manual*, Supreme Grand Lodge of AMORC. Calif. 1918

K. F. Meyer, *The Animal Kingdom, reservoir of human disease*; Ann. Intern, Medicine, 29:326, 1948

F. Fenner, *The Biology of animal viruses*; Academic Press, New York, 1968. Vol. 2.

R. W. Horne, *The Structure of Viruses*; Scientific American, 28:48 1963

D. B. Wilson & R. E. Billingham; *Lymphocytes and Transplantation Immunity*; Advances Immun. 7:189, 1967

Weiser, Myrvik &-Pearsall; *Fundamentals of Immunology*, Lea and Febiger, Philadelphia, 1969

H. Zinsser, *Rats, Lice and History*; Little, Brown & Co., Boston, 1934

H. A. Lechevalier, & M. Solotorovsky, *Three Centuries of Microbiology*, McGraw-Hill Book Co., New York, 1965

G. F. Moore, *Metempsychosis*, Harvard University Press, Cambridge, MA

Moses Goldstein, *Dietary Barbarisms*, Brooklyn, 1926

Edmund Gathercoal, *Pharmacognosy*, Lea & Febiger, Philadelphia, 1936

Ralph Whiteside Kerr, *Herbalism Through the Ages*, Supreme Grand Lodge of AMORC, 1966

Richard Pankhurst, *An Introduction to the Medical History of Ethiopia*, The Red Sea Press, Trenton, NJ 1990

S. Raffel; *Immunity*, Appleton-Century-Crofts, New York, 1961

Stanislas De Rola; *Alchemy: The Secret Art*, 1974

Kurt K. Doberer; *The Goldmakers: Ten Thousand Years of Alchemy*, translated by E. W. Dickes, 1948

Arthur Suzman; *Six Million did Die*, Johannesburg, S. A. 1978

Ra Un Nefer Amen; *Metu Neter, The Great Oracle of Tehuti*, Khamit Corporation, Brooklyn, NY 1990

Yu Lu Kuan; *Alchemy and Immortality*, Samuel Weiser Inc. New York

Neil Powell; *Alchemy: The Ancient Science*, London 1977

Baron Karl Von Reichenbach; *Researches on the Vital Force*, University Books, Secaucus, NJ 1974

P. Stanley Yoder; *African Health and Healing Systems*, Los Angeles, Calif, 1982

Ulrike Sulikowsky; *Eating the Flesh, Eating the Soul*, Paris, 1993

Edith Turner; *Experiencing Ritual. A new interpretation of African Healing*, Philadelphia, 1992

M. Akn Makinde; *African Philosophy, Culture and Traditional Medicine*. Athen, 1988

Philip Ziegler; *The Black Death*, New York, 1990

Samuel L. Epstein; *The Politics of Cancer*, Sierra Books, 1978

Richard LaFond; *Cancer – The Outlaw Cell*, American Chemical Society, 1978

Arnold E. Reif, *Immunity and Cancer in Man.* Marcel Dekker, Inc., New York, 1975

Josef Issels, *Cancer: A Second Opinion.* Hodder & Stoughton, London, 1975

George Ohsawa, *Cancer and the Philosophy of the Far East.* Swan House Publishing Co. Binghamton, NY 1971

Ralph W. Moss, *The Cancer Syndrome.* Grove Press, New York, 1980

Judith Glassman, *The Cancer Survivors.* The Dial Press, New York, 1983

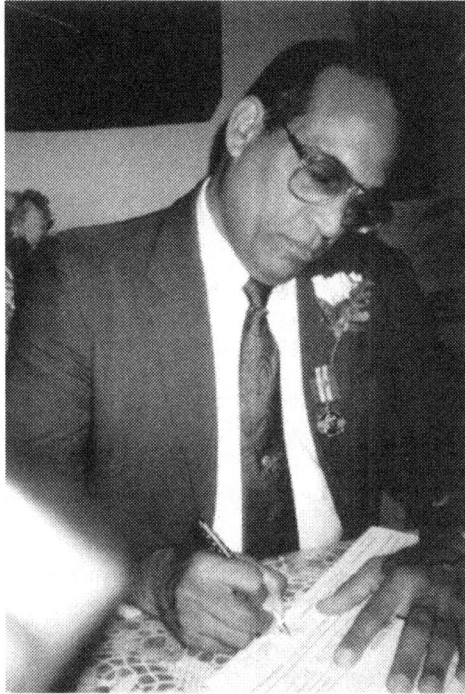

About the Author

Miguel F. Brooks is an Historical and Biblical researcher, lecturer and Public Speaker. A graduate of the Instituto Istmeño in Panamá and Universidad de Carabobo in Venezuela, he holds a B.Sc. Degree in General Science and a Ph.D. in Psychology.

Miguel Brooks has attained unto the Higher Temple Degrees in AMORC, Ancient and Mystical Order of the Rose and the Cross, and in the Rose Croix d'Egypte (Esoteric and Metaphysical Studies) and was awarded the Centenary Gold Medal of the Battle of Adwa by the Ethiopian Crown Council for his work in the field of Ethiopian History and Culture.

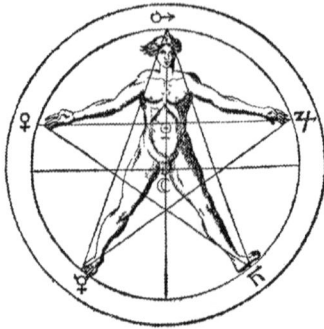

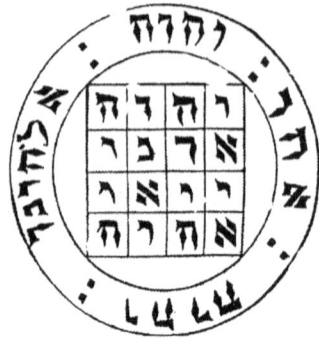

UPCOMING BOOKS BY MIGUEL F. BROOKS

Author of: *"Kebra Nagast" (The Glory of Kings)*
"Negus" (Majestic Tradition of Ethiopia)
"Seeking: THE ALCHEMICAL CURE FOR CANCER"

For Publication

"CANCER ALCHEMY IN JAMAICA" (The Clinical Trials)

In this sequel to "Seeking: The Alchemical Cure for Cancer", the author narrates the daunting challenges faced by his small research team, as they forge ahead in their determination to test the ancient cure for Cancer, that was only available to the aristocracy and nobility of antiquity.

With minimal resources, little help, and operating in total secrecy, these modern day Alchemists conduct a series of clinical trials on terminally ill cancer patients, in order to confirm or deny the safety and efficacy of the exotic "natural" cure for Cancer.

"IN THE MIND OF THE TORTURER"

A readable and explicit journey into the psyche of the torturer, examining the motivations, urges and dark compulsions that fuel his methodical and careful application of exquisitely diabolic tortures. The cognitive processes, the rare emotions and moral dilemmas of the very human "monster of cruelty" are vividly described from his perspective and from within his mind. Revealing and disturbing. Its almost like staring deeply into a mirror...

"IN THE MIND OF THE ATHEIST"

The agonizing, mind-bending philosophical contortions of an ordinary man as he seeks answers to his endless quest in search of an utterly indifferent God. Walk hand - in - hand with a perceptive original thinker as he looks outside for the One that is really within; the One that is truly, only he himself.

"IN THE MIND OF THE SADIST"

The inner workings of the sadistic personality as he contemplates the murky and frightening desires that impels him to seek that familiar, quasi orgasmic thrill, in the intensely agonic pain he inflicts on others.

As he becomes jaded through the many victims of his pathos, he is tempted to experience the pain himself and is gradually transformed into a sadomasochist, endlessly searching for that elusive 'high' where pain and pleasure are intermingled and become one and the same.

184

www.ingramcontent.com/pod-product-compliance
Lightning Source LLC
Chambersburg PA
CBHW031932190326
41519CB00007B/501